MINERAL MIRACLE

MINERAL MIRACLE

STOPPING CARTILAGE LOSS & INFLAMMATION NATURALLY

SHARI LIEBERMAN, PhD, CNS
ALAN XENAKIS, MD, ScD, MPH

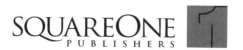
SQUAREONE
PUBLISHERS

COVER DESIGNER: Jacqueline Michelus and Jeannie Tudor
TYPESETTER: Gary A. Rosenberg

The information and advice contained in this book are based upon the research and the personal and professional experiences of the authors. They are not intended as a substitute for consulting with a health care professional. The publisher and authors are not responsible for any adverse effects or consequences resulting from the use of any of the suggestions, preparations, or procedures discussed in this book. All matters pertaining to your physical health should be supervised by a health care professional. It is a sign of wisdom, not cowardice, to seek a second or third opinion.

Square One Publishers
115 Herricks Road
Garden City Park, NY 11040
(516) 535-2010 • (877) 900-BOOK
www.squareonepublishers.com

Library of Congress Cataloging-in-Publication Data

Lieberman, Shari.
  Stopping cartilage loss and inflammation naturally /
Shari Lieberman, Alan Xenakis.
    p. cm.
  Includes bibliographical references and index.
  ISBN 0-7570-0265-X (pbk.)—ISBN 0-7570-0291-9 (hardcover)
  1. Minerals—Therapeutic use. 2. Dietary supplements—Therapeutic use.
3. Minerals in the body. 4. Inflammation—Alternative treatment. 5. Arthritis—
Alternative treatment. 6. Self-care, Health. I. Xenakis, Alan Perry. II. Title.

RM258.5.L56 2006
613.2′85—dc22   2005030349

Printed in Canada

10   9   8   7   6   5   4   3

Contents

Preface

We live in a world in which significant medical and nutritional discoveries are routine. Wondrous findings are published in prestigious medical journals, yet precious few of these discoveries actually eliminate suffering. A major reason for this growing gap between research and practice is the sheer breadth of evolving knowledge, as well mass media's greater comfort in reporting prescription-related breakthroughs than discoveries of therapeutic supplements. The immensity of information about prescription and natural supplements makes it nearly impossible for today's physicians to successfully apply new treatments in a timely and effective fashion. The result is that you may be suffering needlessly even though supporting therapies to prevent or treat your chronic condition exist.

The purpose of this book is to translate and collate the scientific findings on SierraSil into a practical primer that can help you stop or significantly curtail chronic joint and degenerative disease causes and symptoms. To do so, we must erase the barriers that random mountains of data create, and simplify the valuable information you need to have right now.

The majority of chronic human suffering and premature death associated with degenerative disease is avoidable. It is imperative that you take responsibility for directing the key elements of your own care. On average, most practicing physicians can devote only twelve minutes to each patient. You cannot reasonably expect a typical physician to provide you with the time you need for the best care possible. It is up to you, then, to assist your doctor in every way you can as you strive for good health.

History has never seen a time when so much important information has been left by the wayside, unavailable to the patient. But every individual who suffers from the pain of inflammatory disease needs to know about the SierraSil mineral complex. This book provides all the information you require to integrate SierraSil into your treatment regimen.

We cannot overemphasize the importance of educating yourself about the elements involved in your chronic joint and degenerative disease. Patients who are well informed have been found to experience greater success in their health care than passive patients who understand little about their disorders and the treatments used to relieve them. We are confident that when you finish reading this book, you will be able to manage your health care with the minimum prescription medication you need, coupled with the right balance of diet, exercise, and targeted therapeutic supplements. Always keep in mind that health is your best friend, while prescription drugs are simply acquaintances.

Introduction

I t's midnight. You try to fall sleep, but with every toss and turn, the jarring pain in your joints keeps you up. You take a deep breath, go into the bathroom, and grab a bottle of extra-strength aspirin from the medicine cabinet. After taking two (all the while wondering how removing a simple cap from a bottle can hurt so much), you climb back into bed and finally fall asleep. The next thing you know, the alarm rings. You stretch your arm over to shut it off, and as soon as you do, you feel a sharp pain in your shoulder. You get out of bed *very slowly*. As you stand, you begin to shift your weight and the pain seems to move from your shoulder to your back to your knees. You head for the bathroom once again—this time to take your prescribed anti-inflammatory medication. You tell yourself that you'll be fine in thirty minutes or so. But will you?

For millions of Americans, this scenario repeats itself day after day. We have become a nation that is dependent upon drugs. What's most disturbing is that these treatments don't eliminate the cause of our pain. They merely mask the problem by temporarily alleviating the discomfort. And the more drugs we take, the more we rely on them to get us through each day and night.

Fortunately, there is a healthy alternative to this approach—one that not only helps you experience safe and significant joint pain relief from arthritis and other inflammatory conditions, but also addresses the cause. This new natural supplement is called

SierraSil. It is a unique mineral complex that supports the cessation of or noticeably reduces chronic inflammation, which medical researchers now know is one of the primary causes of arthritis and other degenerative illnesses. In the chapters that follow, you will learn about this new natural supplement that is a true gift of the earth. We call it the "mineral miracle."

What constitutes a miracle? If you woke up each day with pain that disrupted your sleep, interfered with your daily routine, increased fatigue, and prevented you from enjoying your favorite activities, you might consider anything that stopped that pain a miracle—whether a pharmaceutical drug or a natural product. Of course, as you will soon see, in the case of drugs, with their inherent array of often-serious side effects, your "prescription miracle" might turn out to be a nightmare.

As health practitioners who emphasize an integrative approach to health care, we combine the best of both conventional and alternative medicine. As researchers who are devoted to learning all we can about safe, natural, and effective nutritional supplements, we are always on the lookout for products and therapies that provide maximum benefit with minimum risk. When we find them, we become excited and eager to share them with our patients and colleagues. It is why we are so grateful to be able to share the SierraSil discovery with you.

If you are reading this book, there's a good chance you are one of the millions of Americans who are turning to natural solutions to address your health concerns. Once part of a small minority, you and others like you now belong to an ever-growing population of health-conscious consumers. According to the latest surveys, more than two-thirds of all Americans now use some form of alternative medicine, with nutritional and herbal therapies being the most popular.

Due to the continued growth and popularity of the natural heath products industry—a trend that began in the 1960s and mushroomed by the early 1990s—it is not uncommon for advertising hype and false claims to be made about so-called "miracle products." That is why we both devote so much of our time investigating such claims and "separating the wheat from the chaff," so that you, the consumer, can be aware of what works and what doesn't. To this end, we both continue to stay abreast of the latest developments in this field, attending and presenting at medical conferences all around the world. We rarely, however, find a product that works as powerfully and effectively as the one we introduce in this book. But before discussing what you will be learning about SierraSil in the chapters that follow, let's examine some of the factors that are causing more and more Americans to turn to natural health products as a solution for their healthcare needs.

THE LIMITATIONS OF CONVENTIONAL MEDICINE

Most proponents of conventional medicine tend to rely too heavily on prescription drugs. According to a report released by the United States Department of Health and Human Services on December 2, 2004, Americans spent $1.6 trillion dollars on health care in 2002, the most recent year for which that data is available. Just how big is that number? In that year alone, we spent three times the amount allocated to rebuild the city of New Orleans and other areas of the Gulf Coast destroyed in 2005 by Hurricane Katrina. Ouch! It gets worse. Health experts estimate that in the very near future, that figure will rise to $2 trillion, which means that more than $5,000 is spent per year for every person in the United States.

During that same year, the deaths caused by heart attack, cancer, and stroke—the nation's three biggest killers—decreased only a miniscule 1 to 3 percent (in spite of lipid-lowering drugs, cancer therapies, and other leading prescription drugs). While any decrease in the death rates of these illnesses is commendable, clearly there is room for vast improvement in the way conventional medicine treats these diseases.

Compounding the problem of conventional medicine's resistance to nondrug treatment options is the prohibitive cost of malpractice insurance premiums, an aging population, and the rise of many chronic and degenerative diseases and conditions. Our colleague Dr. Andrew Weil, clinical professor of internal medicine, as well as founder and director of the Program in Integrative Medicine at the University of Arizona's Health Sciences Center in Tucson, states that approximately 85 percent of the health problems we face as a nation are of a chronic, degenerative nature. Every day, more than one-third of all Americans endure such health conditions as allergy, arthritis, asthma, back pain, chronic fatigue, depression, diabetes, gastrointestinal disorders, headaches, high blood pressure, obesity, and osteoporosis.

As Dr. Weil further points out, conventional medicine, for all of its technical advances and arsenal of pharmaceutical drugs, has no answer for chronic disease. At best, it can offer only temporary relief of symptoms through medication, but it fails to address the underlying causes of such conditions. As a result, people who rely on prescription drugs for relief of chronic pain and suffering must take them indefinitely. Not only can doing so be very expensive, but pain-relieving drugs also carry risks of potentially harmful side effects, even death.

Neither of us is opposed to the sensible use of pharmaceutical drugs, and we won't hesitate to recommend them to our patients if we think they can make a positive difference. However, we both recognize that they are increasingly overused, often without providing the promised results. Most disturbing, in many cases, they result in very serious consequences. Consider the following grim statistic: According to the *Journal of the American Medical Association (JAMA)*, one of the most highly regarded publications in the field of conventional medicine, each and every year in this country, pharmaceutical drugs, *when properly prescribed*, cause the deaths of over 100,000 people, and adverse side effects to millions of others.

NATURAL HEALTH PRODUCTS—A SAFER ALTERNATIVE

While it is true that natural products are not without risk, growing scientific evidence clearly shows that overall they are often far safer than many prescription drugs in a similar category, and they are capable of producing equal or superior results. Although recently, the FDA has raised the alarm on nutritional and herbal health products—a result of the 153 deaths allegedly linked to the herb ephedra—the fact remains that when taken as directed, nutritional supplements are significantly safer than the majority of drugs you and I can purchase over the counter, including aspirin.

Some health experts maintain that you can get all of the nutrition you need from the foods you eat. We respectfully but firmly disagree with this belief for a number of reasons. For starters, as our society's obesity epidemic makes clear, many of us don't make wise food choices. Instead, we rely on unhealthy fast-food meals that are devoid of nutrients.

But even those of us who are committed to eating healthy, and who place a premium on buying and eating organic foods whenever possible, are still at risk of being nutritionally deficient if we rely on diet alone. The reason is that our foods—even those raised organically—no longer contain the same abundance of vitamins, minerals, and other essential elements that were contained in the foods of our ancestors. This erosion of essential food-based nutrients is due primarily to the demineralization of crop soils as a result of commercial farming methods.

And then there are the environmental toxins and pollutants we are exposed to daily. Toxins such as carbon monoxide, sulfur dioxide, hydrocarbons, and second-hand smoke have been linked to a wide variety of health conditions, as well as premature aging and mental decline. Nutritional supplements can play a vital role in counteracting the effects of these toxins.

From our perspective, eating wisely and supplementing your diet with essential nutrients daily is a safe, effective, and inexpensive means of lessening your risk of disease. It's no secret that the vast majority of our holistically inclined professional colleagues agree with us. What is not so well known is that the *Journal of the American Medical Association* does also. In 2002, *JAMA* published an article by Harvard researchers recommending that "all adults take one multivitamin daily." This recommendation was based on a review of thirty years of scientific articles that explored the relationship between nutrients and chronic illness.

Just as telling, a recent survey of dieticians—who, as a class of healthcare providers, perpetuate the belief that all of the nutrients we need are available through a balanced diet—found that nearly

60 percent regularly use nutritional supplements. No doubt they are aware of studies showing how the majority of Americans are deficient in a number of vital nutrients. Some health experts estimate that as many as 80 percent of the US population falls into this category.

Of course, nutritional supplements alone are no panacea for poor health and disease, and they certainly cannot take the place of a healthy well-balanced diet; but the improvements we have seen them make in countless patients are nothing short of remarkable. These enrichments are supported by a growing body of clinical and laboratory results that meet the criteria for scientific peer review publication.

But this doesn't mean you should take nutritional supplements indiscriminately. Nor should you believe the purported benefits of a particular supplement just because its manufacturer or supplier touts them. In the course of reading this book, you will learn how to supplement wisely; discover which vitamins, minerals, and other co-nutrients are essential for good health; and learn the optimal dosage range for each. In addition, you will be introduced to the exciting nutritional product we referred to earlier—the unique mineral compound called SierraSil, which can make a dramatic difference in the way you feel.

WHAT THIS BOOK WILL TEACH YOU

In the chapters that follow, you will learn all about the SierraSil mineral complex. In an effort to present a clear, accurate, and comprehensive picture of this amazing natural supplement, we have included pertinent, interesting, often compelling information that covers such topics as:

✔ The unique role minerals play in your health, how and why they are so vitally important, and which ones you need on a daily basis.

✔ The story of SierraSil's discovery.

✔ The unique blend of minerals in the deposit from which Sierra-Sil is derived.

✔ The scientific clinical studies that have shown SierraSil to be a safe and effective natural aid for significantly reducing the pain of osteoarthritis and other inflammatory conditions.

✔ How SierraSil is able to support the cessation and prevention of cartilage loss—a condition associated with aging and chronic degenerative diseases.

✔ How SierraSil's unique chemical makeup has been clinically shown to suppress the genetic factors that trigger harmful inflammation.

In addition, we reveal the eye-opening marketing role of pharmaceutical drug companies when bringing out new products, and compare them with the role of natural product manufacturers. We discuss the serious side effects resulting from the most common pharmaceutical pain relievers, from aspirin to COX-2 inhibitors. And we provide a proven multifaceted health regimen that you and your loved ones can follow to safely and effectively protect yourself against disease.

If you or someone you know is suffering from chronic joint pain, and you are searching for a solution that can safely stop that pain, not just mask it, the information contained in this book is for you. If you are one of the millions of informed readers who recognize the importance of disease prevention, this book is also for you. Are you ready to learn all about this "mineral miracle" and put it to work? Turn the page and read on.

CHAPTER 1

The Importance of Minerals to Your Health

ave you ever held a rock in your hand and wondered what it was made of? This may seem like a strange question to lead off a chapter in a health book, but it is an important one. Most likely, that rock you held was made of a combination of common minerals. It may have been formed only a few hundred years ago, or it could have been around before there were humans or dinosaurs or even trees. When life first appeared on this planet, it came from the material that was at hand. To a great extent, the earliest living creatures relied on minerals to give their external and internal structures form and to carry on the basic life processes necessary to sustain their existence. Millions of years later, the descendents of these life forms may have become more sophisticated, but they are no less dependent on minerals than were these earliest creatures. Nor are we.

Today, when most people think of nutritional supplements, they immediately think of vitamins. Although vitamins are certainly important to your overall health, as you will see, they alone are not enough to provide your body with all that it requires to maintain good health. Minerals play an equally important role, for without them, vitamins cannot function properly. And, therefore, neither can you.

In this chapter, we will present all the information you need to fully understand why minerals are so important to your health. You will learn what minerals are, how they are classified, and which ones you need on a daily basis. You'll also discover the many body functions in which they play a vital role. Let's begin our exploration of minerals by discussing what they actually are.

WHAT ARE MINERALS?

Minerals are inorganic elements. This means that unlike vitamins, which are organic, minerals cannot be produced, or synthesized, by plants or animals. Rather, minerals come from the earth itself. They are the end products that remain as ash or inorganic residue (such as silica and iron) from the completely decomposed tissues of plants, animals, and humans. Like vitamins, minerals are absolutely essential for your health, and make up between 4 to 5 percent of the adult body weight of humans. Primarily concentrated in the bones, minerals are also found in varying quantities in bodily fluids and tissues. By far, your body's two most abundant minerals are calcium and phosphorus, which together comprise approximately 75 percent of your entire mineral make-up.

Minerals play many vital roles, working synergistically with vitamins, enzymes, hormones, and other nutrient cofactors to regulate literally thousands of your body's biological functions. Proper blood formation, energy production, nerve transmission, and regulation of healthy acid-alkaline balance are among these essential functions. Minerals also support healthy bones and teeth and are required for proper support of the body's overall structure and function.

In addition, minerals play a key role in healthy cell function; they are critical for proper cell regeneration as cells progress through their normal life cycle and are replaced by new, healthy cells. If your body's mineral supply is deficient, there is an increased likelihood that both existing cells and the cells that replace them can become compromised, setting the stage for various chronic and degenerative diseases, including cancer. Scientific research has shown, for example, that the minerals zinc and selenium have anticancer properties, and that certain types of cancer have a greater likelihood of occurring and spreading when these minerals are lacking.

Among the many other vital functions that minerals help your body maintain are proper immune function (zinc, for example, boosts resistance to colds and flu, as well as the recovery time for such conditions), metabolism, cardiovascular function, blood sugar regulation (enhanced by both chromium and selenium), muscle contractions, regulation of fluids, stimulation of growth, formation and maintenance of tissue, and cell permeability, which is essential for the cells' ability to both receive oxygen and nutrients through the cell wall, and to eliminate cellular waste. An adequate mineral supply is also necessary for proper mental and cognitive functioning, as well as sound mental health. Minerals are necessary for detoxification, and for aiding the body in resisting and coping with the daily onslaught of environmental toxins. Overall, minerals are so vitally important to health, that the late Dr. Linus Pauling, two-time winner of the Nobel Prize, said, "You can trace every sickness, every disease, and every ailment to a mineral deficiency."

Since your body cannot produce minerals on its own, it is important that you obtain an adequate daily supply of essential minerals from the foods you eat and through the wise use of supplements. Some health experts claim that eating a healthy diet is all that is required to obtain all the necessary nutrients our bodies need. Current peer review scientific literature does not support such a claim.

Certainly, eating wisely is a vitally important step in achieving and maintaining optimal health. However, with all of the health challenges in today's modern world, a healthy diet alone is not enough to ensure that your body's nutritional requirements are being met. We no longer live in the pristine world of our ancestors, who breathed clean air, drank and bathed in fresh clean water, ate fresh whole foods that were nutrient dense, and lived without the physical and psychological stresses that are so common today. Moreover, even if we are able to regularly eat a balanced diet of organic foods, it would still not be good enough. Compared to what was grown only fifty years ago, today's foods contain far fewer vital nutrients, particularly minerals that our bodies need. Due to commercial farming methods, which have greatly depleted the minerals and other nutrients from the soil, our fruits, vegetables, nuts, seeds, and grains, are lacking the value they once had. This practice of devitalizing soil through modern farming methods, as well as the widespread use of chemical fertilizers, pesticides, and other agents for boosting production yields and preserving harvested foods, began in the early 1900s. By 1936, the soil's loss of nutritional value was already so significant that the United States Senate warned against it in U.S. Senate Document No. 264. In part, this document reads:

> The alarming fact is that foods (fruits, vegetables, and grains) now being raised on millions of acres of land that no longer contains enough of certain minerals are starving us—no matter how much we eat. No man of today can eat enough fruits and vegetables to supply his system with the minerals he requires for perfect health because his stomach isn't big enough to hold them. The truth is that our foods vary enormously in value, and some of them aren't worth eating as food. . . . Our physical well-being is more directly dependent upon the minerals we take into our system than upon calories or vitamins or upon the precise proportions of starch, protein, or carbohydrates we consume.

Since that warning (and in spite of it), the situation has only worsened. Decade after decade, the nutrient value of commercially grown foods has continued a steady decline. This fact was confirmed in a study published in the *Journal of the American College of Nutrition* in December 2004. The study, led by Dr. Donald Davis, a biochemist at the University of Texas at Austin, investigated the effects of modern farming methods on the nutrient content of forty-three garden crops (primarily vegetables, but also including melons and strawberries).

In the study, Dr. Davis and his associates compared the nutritional density of the crops grown in 1999 to the same crops grown in 1950 by examining recorded data from both years. The foods were analyzed individually and as a group. Of the thirteen nutrients evaluated, the results showed that the overall levels of six—protein, calcium, phosphorus, iron, riboflavin, and vitamin C—were present in noticeably higher amounts (as much as 38 percent) in the foods grown in 1950 compared to those grown in 1999.

Commenting on the findings, Dr. Davis said, "We conclude that the most likely explanation was changes in cultivated varieties used today compared to fifty years ago. During those fifty years, there have been intensive efforts to breed new varieties that have greater yield, or resistance to pests, or adaptability to different climates. But the dominant effort is for higher yields. Emerging evidence suggests that when you select for yield, crops grow bigger and faster, but they don't necessarily have the ability to make or uptake nutrients at the same, faster rate.

"Perhaps more worrisome," Dr. Davis added, "would be declines in nutrients we could not study because they were not reported in 1950—magnesium, zinc, vitamin B_6, vitamin E, and dietary fiber, not to mention phytochemicals."

According to health journalist Larry Trivieri, Jr., author of *The American Holistic Medical Association Guide to Holistic Health*, overall "[t]he mineral content of soil used to grow today's group is one-sixth of what it was fifty years ago, due to commercial farming methods. . . . Additional commercial farm production methods, along with shipping and storage procedures, further deprive crops of their nutrient value." Such facts clearly show that relying on healthy diet alone is no longer enough to provide the body with a plentiful supply of the minerals, vitamins, and other essential nutrients it needs each and every day.

Compounding the problem is the fact that millions of Americans rely on the standard American diet of convenience foods, which are far more deficient in minerals and other vital nutrients than fresh, whole foods. Many commercial products, such as breads, muffins, and pastas are typically made from refined white flour, which has been stripped of up to 90 percent of its minerals during the refinement process. Even modern food preparation methods add to the problem. Overcooking vegetables, for example, significantly reduces their nutrient content.

As a result of such practices, government surveys continue to show growing mineral deficiencies within the American populace. For example, an estimated 60 percent of all Americans are deficient in magnesium, while as many as 80 percent lack adequate chromium levels. Overall, recent analyses of the nutrient and supplement intake conducted by the National Institutes of Health (NIH) shows that the vast majority of people, both in the United States and in other affluent Western nations, do not even meet 75 percent of the recommended dietary allowances (RDAs) for many essential minerals. Despite this data, focus on the need for a daily mineral intake that is adequate for optimal health continues to be overlooked, not only by the general public, but by many healthcare professionals.

By contrast, veterinarians, as well as cattle farmers and livestock breeders have long recognized the importance of minerals. It is for this reason that minerals are added to the feed of livestock and mineral salt licks are frequently placed in the fields where these animals roam. These measures not only improve the health of the animals, but they prevent a condition known as *cribbing*—a practice in which animals lick or chew on wood or clay to satisfy their craving for the minerals these items contain. If animals and their caretakers recognize the importance of minerals for good health, shouldn't we do the same and take measures to ensure that we get all the minerals our bodies need?

TYPES OF MINERALS

Minerals are classified according to the percentage of the body's total weight they comprise. Minerals that make up 0.01 percent or more are known as *macrominerals,* while those that make up less are considered *trace minerals,* or *trace elements.* The body needs macrominerals in daily dosages of 100 milligrams or more; microminerals are required in much smaller amounts.

Macrominerals

The primary macrominerals your body needs to ensure good health are calcium, chloride, magnesium, phosphorus, potassium, silicon, sodium, and sulfur. What follows is an overview of the roles each of these minerals plays in the health of your body, as well as a listing of common food sources in which they are found.

Calcium

Calcium is the most plentiful mineral in the human body, with 99 percent found in bone tissue. The remaining 1 percent is used in a variety of other functions, including blood clotting, muscle contraction, and nerve transmission. In addition to healthy teeth and bones, calcium contributes to healthy skin, helps regulate cardiovascular function and blood pressure levels, aids in the metabolism of iron, and is required for proper cell division. During times of growth (especially during adolescence and teenage years), pregnancy, and lactation, the body's need for calcium increases.

Common signs of calcium deficiency include bone problems (most notably osteoporosis and fracture), anxiety, brittle nails, depression, insomnia, muscle cramping and twitching, and diminished nerve function. Your body needs calcium daily, which can be supplied through diet or supplementation. Milk, yogurt, cheese, cottage cheese, dark green leafy vegetables, broccoli, turnip and collard greens, salmon, sardines, shrimp, canned fish, almonds, and Brazil nuts are the best calcium food sources.

It is estimated that the standard American diet supplies only one-third of the daily calcium needed by the body. In addition, calcium supplies can be decreased by a variety of factors, including vitamin D deficiency, gastrointestinal disorders, low stomach acid, stress, lack of exercise, and excessive fat and/or protein intake. The body's ability to absorb calcium can also diminish with age.

Chloride

An essential component of hydrochloric acid (HCl)—a vital stomach digestive acid—chloride also plays a role in regulating the body's acid balance. Chloride is significant in helping the liver eliminate toxins, as well as in transporting carbon dioxide to the lungs for excretion. Among the best food sources of chloride are common table salt, sea salt, seaweeds, celery, lettuce, and tomatoes. The standard American diet, which is characterized by a high salt content, contains more than enough chloride.

Chloride loss can easily occur following bouts of diarrhea or vomiting, as well as during periods of profuse perspiration.

Overall, however, chloride deficiencies are rare, with acid-base imbalances and over-alkalinity of body fluids being the most common symptoms.

Magnesium

Magnesium acts as a muscle relaxant and is also involved in hundreds of enzymatic reactions. Approximately 65 percent of the body's magnesium supply is contained in the bones and teeth, with the second-highest concentration occurring in the muscles. The remaining magnesium can be found in the blood and other bodily fluids.

In addition to its ability to relax smooth and skeletal muscles, magnesium is an important nutrient for the heart, especially in preventing spasms of the coronary arteries, which can result in heart attacks. It is also needed for energy production, the maintenance and repair of cells, healthy cell division, proper nerve transmission, hormone regulation, and the metabolism of proteins and nucleic acids.

Plants that are rich in chlorophyll, particularly dark green vegetables, are the primary food sources of magnesium. Nuts, seeds, legumes, tofu, wheat germ, millet, brown rice, apricots, and avocados are other good sources.

Magnesium deficiency, which is becoming more and more common, is a growing concern. Contributing factors include poor dietary choices, overcooked foods, the overuse of alcohol, and nutrient-poor soil in which foods are grown. Symptoms of magnesium deficiency include depression, fatigue, irregular heartbeat, gastrointestinal disorders, high blood pressure, memory problems, mood swings, impaired motor skills, muscle spasms, nausea, and tetany (numbness, tingling, and/or cramping of the hands, arms, feet, or legs).

Phosphorus

Second to calcium as the body's most abundant mineral, phosphorus is present in every cell of the body, but primarily (approximately 85 percent) in the bones and teeth. Along with contributing to bone and tooth structure, phosphorus helps form DNA and RNA, catalyzes B-complex vitamins, and is involved in cellular communication and numerous enzymatic reactions. It also helps produce energy and increase endurance.

The best food sources of phosphorus are protein foods, such as meats, fish, poultry, eggs, milk, and cheese. Other good sources include nuts, seeds, wheat germ, whole grains, and brewer's yeast. The standard American diet often contains too much phosphorus—carbonated soft drinks alone can have up to 500 milligrams per serving. Too much phosphorus causes a calcium-phosphorus imbalance. This imbalance impairs the body's ability to absorb calcium and increases the amount it draws from the bones.

Due to the fact that phosphorus is contained in all animal foods, phosphorus deficiency is rare among non-vegetarians. However, overuse of antacids, excessive calcium intake, and lack of vitamin D can all result in a deficiency of this mineral. Signs of phosphorus deficiency include anxiety, loss of appetite, impaired bone growth, loss of bone mass, irritability, muscle cramps, dizziness, and general weakness.

Potassium

Along with chloride and sodium, potassium is an *electrolyte* or *essential body salt* that conducts electric currents throughout the body. Approximately 98 percent of the body's potassium supply is contained within the cell walls, where it regulates water and acid-alkaline balance. Potassium is vital to cellular integrity and fluid balance, and plays an important role in nerve function. It also helps metabolize proteins and carbohydrates, aids in energy production, and helps regulate heartbeat. Optimum food sources of potassium include fresh vegetables and fruits, with bananas being a particularly rich source. Whole grains, seeds, nuts, wheat germ, salmon, and sardines are also good dietary sources.

Potassium deficiencies are fairly common, particularly among people over fifty-five and those suffering from chronic diseases or conditions such as diabetes. Diarrhea, fasting, and the overuse of diuretics and laxatives all contribute to potassium loss. Common symptoms of potassium deficiency include arrhythmia, depression, fatigue, mood swings, high blood pressure, hyperglycemia, impaired growth, and unhealthy changes in the nervous system. Compounding the risk of such symptoms is the fact that most Americans consume far more sodium than potassium each day, creating an imbalance of these two minerals and exacerbating potassium deficiency.

Silicon

Silicon is the most abundant mineral in the earth's crust. In the body, it is most commonly found in bone, blood vessels (arteries), cartilage, collagen, tendons and other connective tissue, eyes, and nails. The body requires silicon for tissue strength and stability, and healthy bones, skin, hair, and nails. Due to its ability to penetrate deep into the tissues to aid in the elimination of stored cellular toxins, silicon is considered a detoxification mineral. Recent research also suggests that it may play a role in cardiovascular health (as a protective agent against heart disease and hardening of the arteries), tissue repair and healing, and stamina and endurance levels.

Silicon is a primary component of plant fibers. Since its levels in the soil are becoming more and more depleted, there is speculation and concern that this mineral deficiency may affect the inherent structure of plants. Silicon is also lost during food processing methods. Common signs of silicon deficiency include brittle nails; osteoporosis; tendonitis, and weak, malformed, or calcified bones.

The hulls of oats, rice, and wheat are the most abundant food sources of silicon. It is also found in alfalfa, avocados, cucumbers, lettuce, onions, and strawberries, as well as many dark green leafy vegetables, such as dandelion greens. The herbs comfrey, horsetail, and nettle are other good silicon sources.

Sodium

Like phosphorus, sodium is present in all of the body's cells. It is also contained in the blood and other bodily fluids. Approximately 60 percent of the body's sodium content is found in extra-cellular fluids (those outside the cells); about 10 percent is contained within the cells, and the remainder is in the bones. Like potassium, sodium helps maintain the body's fluid balance both inside and outside the cells, thereby regulating the body's acid-base balance. It also helps transport carbon dioxide, and plays a significant role in muscle contraction and nerve transmission. In addition, sodium is involved in the production of hydrochloric acid. Sodium plays a helpful role in transporting amino acids to the cells through the bloodstream.

Nearly all foods have some amount of sodium, with seafood, beef, and poultry containing particularly high levels. The primary dietary source of sodium is table salt, although most canned and processed foods also contain significant amounts.

Chronic sodium deficiency is rare, although loss of this mineral can occur due to excessive diarrhea, vomiting, profuse perspiration resulting from strenuous activity, and the overuse of diuretics. Deficiency symptoms include dehydration, low blood pressure, muscle cramping and twitching, and muscle weakness. Problems related to excessive sodium intake are far more common, and often affect people who eat the standard American diet. The body's reaction to too much sodium can lead to high blood pressure and premenstrual syndrome (PMS), among other conditions.

Sulfur

Sulfur is found in all cells and body tissues, especially those with high protein content. The body's total sulfur content is about the same as its potassium content. Sulfur is necessary for the formation of collagen, and is involved in the synthesis of protein. Because it helps maintain healthy hair, skin, and nails, sulfur is sometimes referred to as the "beauty mineral." Sulfur also plays a role in a number of enzymatic reactions, and contributes to the process of cellular respiration. It is necessary for proper brain function, and vital to the cells' ability to utilize oxygen most effectively. Sulfur helps maintain joint health and protects against the development of arthritis. An adequate supply of this mineral also helps ensure the body's detoxification processes, including its proper elimination of waste.

The best food sources of sulfur are those high in protein, such as eggs, fish, legumes, meat, milk, and poultry. Good plant food sources include Brussels sprouts, cabbage, garlic, onions, and turnips.

Common signs of sulfur deficiency include eczema, dermatitis, and brittle hair and nails. Poor hair and nail growth are other signs.

Nutrient Toxicity and Bioavailability

If you are concerned that taking nutritional supplements can have toxic results, please keep in mind that generally, when nutritional supplements are taken as directed, they are less toxic than most over-the-counter drugs, including aspirin. Furthermore, in order to reach toxicity, you would have to really abuse the supplements by taking massive quantities and for prolonged periods of time. In fact, there are virtually no confirmed records of serious adverse side effects resulting from normal healthy people taking vitamin or mineral supplementation when taken according to their recommended daily dosage. However, if you have an existing medical condition, it is always prudent to check with your physician before taking any supplement.

Another consideration when taking nutritional supplements is their *bioavailability,* which is their capacity for absorption and, therefore, utilization by the body. Certain elements are not bioavailable; their uptake by the body is dependent on a variety of factors. For instance, in order to be utilized properly, vitamins and minerals must be taken in conjunction with other elements, and in the right proportions. Take the mineral calcium, for example. For optimal effectiveness, calcium supplements should be taken with magnesium and vitamin D, as these three nutrients work together to enhance each other's absorption and utilization in the body. Calcium and magnesium are also found together, along with vitamins and other minerals, in nutrient-dense foods. In a perfect world, we would be able to get most of these nutrients through diet—just like our ancestors did. Unfortunately, today's environmental conditions make this impossible.

Other factors that can affect nutrient bioavailability include physical exercise (studies have shown that exercise may help improve the absorption of certain minerals and vitamins), any medications being taken, and the physiological, biochemical, and hormonal characteristics of the person taking the supplements.

Trace Minerals

There are ten officially recognized *essential* trace minerals your body needs for optimal health. They are chromium, cobalt, copper, iodine, iron, manganese, molybdenum, selenium, vanadium, and zinc. Additional trace elements that are not considered essential, but are still believed to contribute to good health include boron, lithium, nickel, and strontium.

What follows is an overview of the common benefits provided by these trace minerals along with their best food sources.

Boron

Because of the role it plays in maintaining healthy bones, boron is considered by some health experts to be an essential trace mineral. Boron is concentrated primarily in the parathyroid glands, where it aids in the metabolism and utilization of calcium. It also helps regulate the body's magnesium and phosphorus balance, as well as ensure proper functioning of the endocrine system, which produces and regulates hormones. Boron improves the body's ability to utilize vitamin D, and is important for proper acid-alkaline balance.

No symptoms of boron deficiency have been identified, but because boron is significant in the metabolism of calcium and prevention of bone loss, a deficiency may result in osteoporosis, arthritis, and hypertension.

Boron's primary food sources include leafy green vegetables and fruits, such as apples, grapes, and pears. Nuts and legumes are also good sources. Regular consumption of these foods helps ensure adequate intake of boron, while an unhealthy diet of refined fast foods can lead to a deficiency.

Chromium

Chromium is an essential component of glucose tolerance factor (GTF), which enhances insulin function. This makes chromium vital for proper carbohydrate metabolism and the regulation of blood sugar levels. By improving the body's ability to transport glucose into the cells, chromium and GTF are also important for energy production. Research suggests that chromium may also be useful for regulating the body's cholesterol levels.

Chromium deficiency is quite common in the United States due to mineral-depleted soil and the country's overconsumption of refined and processed foods. Some researchers estimate that as many as half of all Americans do not obtain enough chromium from their diets. Teenagers in particular tend to be deficient in this essential trace mineral due to their reliance on fast foods. In addition, many people have problems absorbing chromium, particularly as they get older.

Among the most common symptoms of chronic chromium deficiency are diabetes-like blood sugar problems and hypoglycemia. Anxiety, fatigue, and impaired cholesterol metabolism are also associated with a lack of dietary chromium. Chromium deficiency is believed to contribute to decreased growth in children and teenagers, as well as slower than normal healing times following injury or surgery.

One of the best dietary sources of chromium is brewer's yeast. Other good sources include whole grain breads and cereals, wheat germ, eggs, meats (especially beef), and shellfish.

Cobalt

A component of vitamin B_{12}, cobalt plays an essential role in the production and healthy functioning of red blood cells and assists in the overall health of other body cells. It aids in nerve health and neuromuscular functions, helps the body produce energy, and contributes to proper digestion. In addition, cobalt is involved in many enzymatic reactions.

Symptoms of cobalt deficiency are similar to those caused by a lack of vitamin B_{12}. The most common signs include pernicious anemia, nausea, loss of appetite, and nerve damage. Lack of cobalt can also contribute to the body's diminished ability to utilize vitamin B_{12}.

The best food sources of cobalt include beet greens, cabbage, figs, legumes, milk, spinach, liver, fish, and sea vegetables.

Copper

Present in all body tissues, copper is found primarily in the liver and brain. It aids in the manufacture of collagen and hemoglobin, and, along with iron, is necessary for the synthesis of oxygen in red blood cells. Copper acts as an antioxidant, helping to protect against free radical damage, a major contributing factor to premature aging and many chronic, degenerative conditions and diseases, including cancer. Copper also plays a role in bone formation and healing processes, helps to increase iron absorption, and plays an important role in a variety of enzymatic reactions.

Mild copper deficiency is fairly common among the general population. Symptoms include anemia, dermatitis, diarrhea, edema, fatigue, impaired collagen production, labored respiration, tissue and blood vessel damage, and skeletal defects.

Dark green leafy vegetables, eggs, organ meats, poultry, shellfish, and whole grain breads and cereals are among the richest food sources of copper. Beans, dried peas, and nuts, including almonds, Brazil nuts, hazelnuts, pecans, and walnuts are other good sources.

Iodine

Iodine is essential for proper functioning of the thyroid gland. It is a necessary part of the thyroid hormones, which help regulate the body's metabolism and energy production, physical growth, nervous system functioning, circulation, and metabolism. These hormones also helping ensure that the cells of the body receive enough oxygen.

Since thyroid hormones play a role in all body functions, iodine is of vital importance to overall health; yet deficiency of this trace mineral is estimated to affect at least 200 million people worldwide, due primarily to depleted soil conditions. Goiter (swelling of the thyroid) and hypothyroidism (low levels of thyroid hormones) are the classic results of iodine deficiency. Common symptoms include fatigue and listlessness, decreased libido, depression, weight gain, and impaired metabolism.

Iodized salt, fish, shellfish, and sea vegetables, particularly seaweed, are the richest food sources of iodine. Be aware that, when eaten raw and in large quantities, certain vegetables (Brussels sprouts, cabbage, cauliflower, turnips, kale, and spinach) and fruits (peaches and pears) can block the uptake of iodine. These healthy foods should be eaten cooked and in limited amounts, especially by those with underactive thyroids.

Iron

Present in all the cells of the body (usually in combination with protein), iron has the primary function of manufacturing hemoglobin, which is responsible for transporting oxygen from the lungs throughout the body. Iron is also necessary for healthy immune function and energy production. Research suggests it may also play a role in protecting cells and tissues from damage due to oxidation.

Women, especially during their childbearing years, require more iron than men, particularly during pregnancy and menstruation. Approximately 10 percent of all women in the Western world are believed to be iron deficient. Children and the elderly are also prone to iron deficiency. Anemia, a compromised immune system, and/or learning disabilities can be the result. Common symptoms of iron deficiency include dizziness, fatigue, headaches, and impaired sleep.

Among the best food sources of iron are beef and organ meats, brewer's yeast, kelp, molasses, dark green leafy vegetables, legumes, oysters, and sardines.

Lithium

Lithium plays a role in stabilizing serotonin levels. This, in turn, helps to stabilize moods, aid in sleep, and balance brain and nervous system functions. Lithium has also been shown to increase white blood cell count, thereby increasing immune function. Some researchers even speculate that this mineral acts as an anticancer agent.

For many decades, a medicinal form of lithium called *lithium carbonate* has been used to stabilize the extreme mood swings experienced by those with bipolar disorder. It has also been effective in treating insomnia, hyperactivity, and mental delusion. In some instances, lithium carbonate has also proven helpful in the treatment of alcoholism. Not only does it decrease the desire for alcohol, but it also appears to help people feel optimistic and have a more positive outlook on life.

The most common sign of lithium deficiency is chronic depression. Lithium is not found in most foods, although it is contained in sugar cane and seaweed.

Manganese

Manganese supports a variety of enzymatic functions in the body, including the metabolism of proteins and carbohydrates. Required for cholesterol and fatty acid synthesis, as well as the formation of collagen, manganese is essential for proper brain function and the overall health of the nervous system. It is needed for normal growth and development, and for the mending of bones and connective tissue.

Symptoms of manganese deficiency include dizziness, hearing problems, poor blood sugar control, memory loss, convulsions, poor muscle coordination and weakness.

The best food sources of manganese are green leafy vegetables, especially spinach; avocados; seaweed; nuts and seeds, especially pecans and hazelnuts; organ meats; oatmeal; and whole grains, particularly buckwheat and whole wheat.

Molybdenum

Along with copper, molybdenum is necessary for the proper utilization of iron and the metabolism of carbohydrates. It promotes healthy cell function and helps the body detoxify potentially toxic sulfites, which are commonly used to preserve food. Because molybdenum is found in most foods, deficiency is uncommon; however, those whose regular diets are high in processed and refined foods are at risk.

Symptoms of molybdenum deficiency include anemia, and mouth and gum disorders. Those who are deficient in this mineral also have a greater risk of dental caries. On the other hand, excessive molybdenum intake can result in elevated uric acid levels and the development of gout-like symptoms. The best dietary sources of molybdenum are leafy green vegetables, beans, peas, legumes, and whole grains.

Nickel

Although nickel is not considered a essential trace mineral, many health experts believe it is. One of the most common minerals in the earth's crust, nickel is also found in many foods. In the body, nickel is most highly concentrated in nucleic acids, especially ribonucleic acid (RNA). It helps in the formation of protein and the metabolism of glucose. Nickel is also an important trace mineral for women who are breastfeeding because of the role it plays in the production of *prolactin*—a hormone that is vital for stimulating breast milk secretion.

Nickel is found in most plant foods, with hazelnuts and walnuts as particularly good sources. The grains barley, buckwheat, corn, and oats are good sources of nickel, as are most vegetables, beans, and legumes. Pears and bananas are the best fruit sources of nickel. By contrast, meats and seafood contain relatively low levels of this mineral.

Selenium

In recent decades, selenium has become recognized as an important mineral that is capable of performing many of the same antioxidant functions as vitamin E. Most important, selenium protects the body's immune system by preventing the formation of free radicals. When combined with vitamin E, it helps maintain a healthy heart, minimizing the risk of cardiovascular disease. In addition, selenium aids liver function, assists in the manufacture of proteins, helps neutralize heavy metals and other toxic substances, and acts as an anti-carcinogen.

Selenium deficiency can result in an increased risk of cancer, cardiovascular disease, high blood pressure, and stroke. Common symptoms include fatigue, skin problems, and infections.

The best dietary sources of selenium are whole grains, soybeans, and Brazil nuts that are grown in selenium-rich soil. Seafood, meats, and organ meats from animals whose diets were high in this mineral are other rich sources. Fruits and vegetables typically contain low levels of selenium, although broccoli, onions, and tomatoes are good sources (again, depending on the soil in which they are grown).

Strontium

Strontium helps to maintain the structure of the body's cells. It is also believed to play a role in maintaining healthy bones and teeth—it helps prevent tooth decay and soft bones. Interestingly, according to research, an adequate supply of strontium may help protect against radiation poisoning from radioactive strontium, which is a byproduct of nuclear fission.

Strontium deficiency can result in dental caries, bone pain, and osteoporosis. Although strontium is found in most plant foods and dairy products, the levels are low.

Vanadium

Vanadium was recognized for its importance to health as early as 1932, when it was cited as a treatment for diabetes and neurasthenia—a disorder associated with a weak or exhausted nervous system that can result in anxiety, fatigue, irritability, and/or localized pains that have no apparent physical cause. More recently, vanadium has been shown to help lower cholesterol levels and aid the body in metabolizing fats.

Although there are no proven symptoms of vanadium deficiency, some scientific researchers speculate that a lack of this mineral can increase the risk of both cancer and heart disease. Vanadium has also been shown to improve blood sugar control and insulin resistance.

While vanadium is found in many foods, generally, it is not contained in significant levels. The best dietary sources, however, are unsaturated fats and vegetable oils, as well as the foods these oils come from, such as corn, olives, and sunflower seeds. Buckwheat, cabbage, carrots, dill, eggs, green beans, oats, parsley, radishes, and rice are other sources. Among seafood varieties, herring and oysters contain vanadium. Most multi-mineral supplements do not contain this trace mineral, making supplementation difficult.

Zinc

One of the most important mineral nutrients, zinc is necessary for the proper functioning of more than 200 enzymatic reactions in the body. It acts as a powerful antioxidant and detoxifier, and is essential for healthy body tissues, growth and development, regulation of insulin, and proper immune function. In men, zinc is important for prostate gland health. In addition, it plays a vital role in cellular membrane structure and function, and helps maintain adequate levels of vitamin A in the body.

Symptoms of zinc deficiency include dermatitis, fatigue, susceptibility to infections, hair loss, impaired immune function, loss of appetite, diminished libido, and prostate conditions.

The best food sources of zinc include beef and other meats; poultry, particularly dark meat; fish and other seafood, especially oysters; and eggs. Whole grain breads and cereals, nuts, legumes, and brewer's yeast are other good sources. Because they avoid animal foods, vegetarians have a tendency to experience zinc deficiency. Eating plenty of whole grains and other plant sources that contain zinc can help prevent this deficiency. It's important to note that zinc can interfere with copper absorption, therefore zinc and copper supplements should be taken apart from each other.

CLAY—THE LITTLE KNOWN HEALING MINERAL

Although the concept of ingesting clay may not seem appealing, certain forms have been used for centuries for their health benefits. Clay is a generic term for an aggregate of hydrous silicate particles less than four micrometers in diameter. It consists of a variety of phyllosilicate minerals, rich in silicon and aluminium oxides and hydroxides. Clays are generally formed by the chemical weathering of silicate-bearing rocks by carbonic acid, but some are formed by hydrothermal activity.

One form in particular called *smectite* has been valued for its many curative properties by over two hundred cultures around the world. And a number of indigenous healing traditions recommend consuming a small amount (about one teaspoon) every day to help maintain good health. Surprisingly, this is a little-known fact in the United States, and yet, the practice of eating clay is so common, it has a medical name—*geophagy*. Geophagy is the eating of an earthy substance, and refers not only to the ingesting of clay, but also to the consumption of chalk or earth.

How the healing properties of clay came to be discovered remains unknown. Perhaps our ancestors instinctively recognized its healing abilities through observation—certain animals eat clay, and pregnant women sometimes experience an instinctual desire to eat small handfuls of this substance during their pregnancies. No matter how its healing capabilities were discovered, clay has been used for health purposes by cultures throughout the world for millennia. The healer-priests in ancient Egypt prescribed it as a purifying agent, not only for the living, but also for their dead. Clay was used in the mummification process to ensure that the departing pharaohs might enter the next world in a state of health and purity. Clay is also mentioned in the medical texts of ancient India as part of the healing apothecary of *Ayurveda*—India's traditional system of medicine.

In the Western world, the recorded use of clay for medicinal purposes extends back nearly two thousand years to the time of Pliny the Elder (23–79 CE), who was considered the greatest natural healer of the Roman Empire. He devoted an entire chapter to the many healing properties of clay in *Natural History,* his most famous text. Dioscorides (40–90 CE), the physician to Nero who also accompanied the Roman armies on their military campaigns throughout Europe and Asia Minor, also wrote of clay's healing virtues in his five-volume treatise *De Materia Medica.* The first systematic pharmacopoeia ever written in the West, *De Materia Medica* catalogued over 600 medicinal plants and more than 1,000 different medications. Galen (130–200 CE), the famed Greek physician and writer, also wrote of clay's value as a medicinal agent, recommending it both internally as a purifier and externally as a poultice. Avicenna (980–1037 CE), the leading physician and philosopher of his time in the Muslim world, extolled clay's ability to heal.

During the eighteenth century, Germany saw a revival of clay's use for healing thanks to naturopathic healers like Sebastian Kneipp (1821–1897). A Bavarian priest, Kneipp also popularized the use of hydrotherapy (therapeutic hot and cold water baths) to improve health. In the early twentieth century, based on Kneipp's teachings, German physicians used clay to successfully treat Asiatic cholera, an infectious disease of the small intestine. During War World One, French, German, and Russian soldiers were given clay along with their food rations. Physicians from all three nations used clay both internally and externally to successfully treat cases of diarrhea, dysentery, food poisoning, and wound infection, which were rampant during the war. In fact, several regiments of French soldiers reported that clay taken with mustard kept them free of dysentery altogether. Among the famous personalities who have recommended eating clay for health include Mahatma Gandhi and jazz composer and musician Charles Mingus, who made it a point to eat a handful of clay-containing dirt each and every day—a practice he said was part of his family tradition.

Clay's healing properties are also well known to animals. According to Ray Knishinsky, author of *The Clay Cure*, many animals lick clay on a regular basis, probably as an instinctual recognition of the minerals it contains. If injured, animals will often roll

Healing Uses of Clay

Regular daily consumption of small amounts of healing clay, as well as the use of clay poultices, baths, and/or facials, have been reported to help a variety of health conditions, including allergies; anemia; arthritis and rheumatism; chronic fatigue syndrome; and gastrointestinal disorders, such as constipation, diarrhea, diverticulitis, food poisoning, bad breath, hemorrhoids, irritable bowel syndrome, and nausea. Other conditions that benefit from healing clay include gum disease; hay fever; headaches; liver conditions, including mild cases of cirrhosis and hepatitis; menstrual cramps; prostate problems; ulcers; and skin conditions, such as acne, eczema, and hives.

Due to its rich supply of *diastases*—a class of enzymes that helps keep the blood rich with oxygen and free of impurities—healing clay is believed to be beneficial to the cardiovascular system. (Blood that contains impurities can eventually contribute to heart disease.) In addition, because of clay's negative charge, clay particles are able to neutralize dangerous free radicals, which cause cellular damage and accelerate aging. The use of clay to safeguard cardiovascular function dates back to ancient Persia and Arabia, where people were encouraged to ingest clay in order to strengthen their hearts.

around in clay beds to soothe their symptoms. Knishinsky also reports that rats will instinctively eat clay when they are poisoned, an indication of clay's ability to neutralize toxins.

How Clay Works as a Healing Agent

The healing properties of smectite and some other healing clays are due to two equally important properties—adsorption and absorption. *Adsorption* is a process in which a solid (clay, in this case) attracts other substances to stick to its surface. When healing clay is ingested and moves through the gastrointestinal tract, it quickly attracts toxins, which adhere to the clay and eventually pass from the body. This attraction occurs because the clay particles carry a negative electrical charge, while the toxins carry a positive charge.

In many indigenous cultures around the world, eating clay is recommended to ensure a healthy pregnancy. For years, anthropologists and sociologists have reported instances of expectant mothers eating mouthfuls of clay, chalk, and dirt. Researchers John Hunter and Oscar Horst witnessed this practice in El Salvador, and reported on it for the National Geographic Society in 1989. They recounted one experience in which they were at a local Salvadoran market and observed a woman and her adult daughter browsing among the clay tablets, which are widely available there as an aid for healthy pregnancy. When asked if the clay tablets really worked, the older woman enthusiastically replied, "Of course they do; I have eight children!"

So what makes ingesting clay so helpful during pregnancy? According to healers of indigenous cultures, it is believed to enhance fertility and help detoxify a woman's body, allowing the fetus to develop in a healthier internal environment. Clay is also used to prevent or minimize morning sickness, safeguard against miscarriage, and ease labor pains. When babies are poorly positioned inside the womb, making natural childbirth more challenging, native midwives often apply clay poultices to the pregnant woman's belly throughout the last month of pregnancy. Once their child is born, new mothers often continue to eat clay and rub it on their breasts to ensure healthy lactation as they nurse their newborns.

When clay particles come in contact with toxins, they are drawn to each other in the same way a magnet attracts metal filings. Winemakers and brewers of beer and cider recognize this characteristic of clay. They add small amounts to their brews to attract positively charged impurities, which are then removed. In the human body, a similar process occurs when clay is ingested. Since clay is not digestible, the toxins it attracts are held on its surface until they are both expelled from the body during elimination. Only substances that are active or alive are capable of adsorption. For this reason, healing clay is considered "alive."

The action through which a certain substance makes its way into another substance is called *absorption*—the other important property of clay. Through this process, which is much slower than adsorption, certain toxins are pulled beneath the clay's surface. As the toxins are absorbed, the clay expands. This enables the absorption of toxins that are far greater in size than the ingested clay particles.

Healing clay's adsorbent and absorbent qualities make it an excellent substance for purifying the gastrointestinal tract safely and easily. Research has shown that in addition to helping neutralize and eliminate toxins, including heavy metals, herbicides, and pesticides, clay is also capable of absorbing free radicals, viruses, and various types of microscopic parasites. Healing clay can be an important weapon for protecting and restoring immunity and healthy gastrointestinal function.

CONCLUSION

As you have seen in this chapter, minerals are essential for maintaining good health and preventing illness. But a healthy diet alone is not enough to ensure that your body is getting all of the minerals it needs on a daily basis. Given the depleted nutrient content of our nation's soil, as well as today's commercial farming and food preservation methods, the minerals contained in crops are nowhere near optimal.

Given that food is simply not enough to supply your body with the nutrients it needs, we recommend a sensible supplementation program. And as a key element of that program, we strongly encourage—in support of chronic disease treatment—a unique supplement called SierraSil. Containing many of the minerals (including healing clay) you need for good health, SierraSil supplies many of them in a way that your body is able to absorb and utilize best. In the next chapter, you will learn all about this exciting compound, including how it was discovered.

CHAPTER 2

The SierraSil Discovery

Within the last three hundred years, the discoveries of various "natural cures"—from the use of vitamin C-rich limes for treating scurvy to the practice of doctors washing their hands before examining patients—have taken literally decades or longer to gain acceptance by the established medical community. Typically, these types of breakthroughs faced an initial barrage of ridicule and skepticism, because disbelievers inherently felt that such simple treatments would not be effective. Yet, in spite of any roadblocks they faced, these "miracle cures" actually worked, eventually leading to their acceptance.

Unfortunately, roadblocks within the medical community still exist and continue to hold back important discoveries of natural products for good health. Among these products is SierraSil. Called the "mineral miracle," SierraSil is a nutritional supplement that—as demonstrated through significant scientific research—has safely and notably supported the reduction of inflammation in the body, and significantly relieved the pain of arthritis. In this chapter, you will learn all about the SierraSil mineral deposit, including how it was discovered and the scientific research that has proven its efficacy—without adverse side effects. But first, consider the following: Why does it typically take so long for the American public, as well as their doctors, to become aware of the benefits that nutritional supplements can provide, while there is near-instant popularity of new pharmaceutical drugs as soon as they enter the marketplace? Let's begin this chapter by taking a closer look at this disturbing truth.

NUTRITIONAL SUPPLEMENT ROADBLOCKS

There is no question that nutritional supplements have, over the last few decades, become an increasingly popular healthcare choice among American consumers. By some estimates, as many as 70 percent of all Americans use some form of nutritional supplementation as part of their overall health maintenance program. Vitamin and mineral supplements are the most popular choices in this area. Yet, the medical establishment had long questioned their validity in supporting the treatment of a wide host of disorders, despite the fact that many of these supplements had voluminous scientific research backing their use. Newly discovered natural products tend to meet the same resistance, which, in turn, prevents them (and their benefits) from reaching those who need them most. Let's examine some of the reasons these benefits have taken so long to garner both awareness and acceptance.

The Long Road to Public Awareness

Vitamin C was discovered in the early twentieth century by Albert von Szent-Gyorgi, who received the Nobel Prize in physiology and medicine for his discovery in 1937. In the 1950s, vitamin C was championed by two-time Nobel Prize recipient Linus Pauling, PhD, who staunchly advocated its supplementation in daily dosages that were well beyond the standard recommended dietary allowance (RDA) of 60 milligrams that had been proposed by Szent-Gyorgi.

At the age of ninety-two, one year before he died, Dr. Pauling was interviewed by health journalist Larry Trivieri, Jr. During that interview, Dr. Pauling shared his belief that a daily vitamin C regimen ". . . is one of the easiest steps anybody can take to help ensure good health."

Today, Dr. Pauling is considered one of the most accomplished biochemists and molecular biologists who ever lived; but for years, most mainstream scientists, researchers, and conventional physicians ridiculed his advocacy of vitamin C. His claims about the vitamin, including its ability to boost immunity and protect against infection, as well as its potent antioxidant properties, have only recently come to be widely accepted. Now, vitamin C supplements, which are sold in dosages ranging from 500 to 1,000 milligrams, are readily available in health food stores, pharmacies, and even grocery stores.

During his interview with Dr. Pauling, Larry Trivieri brought up the subject of nutritional supplementation's struggle with acceptance. He asked Dr. Pauling why he felt the recommendations he had been making about vitamin C since the 1950s had not become widely accepted until decades later. Dr. Pauling explained that, as a nutritionally oriented researcher, every year he was in the habit of reading literally thousands of scientific studies that touted the benefits of nutrients. The vast majority of those studies, however, were not published in the major mainstream medical journals most doctors depend on for the latest medical news. As another interesting point, Dr. Pauling believed that even if the studies had been published in those journals, most doctors would not have read them anyway. He felt that, in general, doctors don't have the time to keep up with the scientific research like he did; they are far too busy treating patients and then making time to be with their families. Is it any wonder that it takes so long for physicians to become aware of a nutrient's potential health benefits?

The Land-of-Plenty Myth

Although an increasing number of conventional physicians are recognizing the benefits of nutritional supplements and recommending them to their patients, others still fail to acknowledge their worth. It's not that they don't believe in the benefits of nutrients; they simply don't believe supplementation is necessary. This attitude stems from the myth that we can meet all of our daily nutritional requirements by eating a well-balanced diet—a myth that is still taught in most medical schools.

The majority of medical doctors are not taught the therapeutic and preventive aspects of using dietary supplements, with the exception of perhaps calcium and vitamin D for osteoporosis.

Most, for example, are still unaware that at least 60 percent of Americans are deficient in magnesium and as many as 80 percent are deficient in chromium. They are taught very little, if at all, about sound eating principles and how to improve one's lifestyle and diet. Those doctors and other healthcare providers who encourage nutrition and other natural modalities in their practice have often gone to great lengths to educate themselves through conferences, continuing education, scientific literature, and other venues.

In Chapter 1, we cited a number of reasons that diet alone does not supply all of the nutrients our body needs. For starters, many people rely on the standard American diet of processed convenience foods, which are stripped of beneficial nutrients during the refining process and/or through cooking techniques. Furthermore, modern farming methods, including the use of chemical fertilizers and pesticides, have robbed the soil of the rich concentrations of the vital minerals it once contained. This results in crops that also contain significantly reduced levels of nutrients compared to those eaten by our ancestors. Once fruits, vegetables, and grains are harvested, they are commonly treated with chemical preservatives or undergo irradiation methods to extend their shelf life.

All of these factors add to the compromised quality of the foods we eat. But that's not all. What follows are some additional reasons that diet alone is not enough to meet our daily nutritional requirements:

■ **Harvesting and preparation methods.** The nutritional value of all types of produce starts to diminish immediately after they are picked and harvested. Unless they are fresh from the garden, fruits and vegetables found in grocery stores or produce markets are likely to be weeks or even months old—and this is true of organic produce, as well. Once they are picked, crops must be stored. Then they are shipped out, which can mean transportation to the next town, the next state, or completely across the country. When they have reached their final destination, they will have to be stored again until they are sold. Each of these steps adds to a product's age and, therefore, to the

depletion of its nutrient content. Exposure to fertilizers, preservatives, herbicides, and various forms of processing further
compromises its value. Even the simple act of cutting a piece of
fruit or slicing a vegetable continues to reduce its vitamin and
mineral content, as does cooking it in temperatures above 110°
Fahrenheit.

■ **Poor bioavailability.** Most people, including many physicians
and other healthcare practitioners, are unaware that a significant portion of many foods we eat is not bioavailable—our bodies cannot absorb it properly. For example, approximately 40
percent of the vitamin C contained in fresh-squeezed orange
juice is biologically inactive and, therefore, unable to be used by
the body. Similarly, although a cup of green cabbage contains
over 50 percent of the daily recommended dietary intake (RDI)
allowance of vitamin C (33 milligrams), more than half of that
amount will not be properly absorbed if the cabbage is eaten
raw. Lightly steaming cabbage is best for maximizing the
bioavailability of the vitamin C it contains. Keep in mind that
overcooking destroys the nutrients contained in all vegetables
and fruits.

■ **Caloric restriction.** A significant portion of the American population struggles with weight issues, including obesity. As a
result, we tend to be a society of dieters; limiting calorie intake
is a common practice for shedding pounds. Most popular
weight-loss diets typically advise a daily total intake of 1,500
calories or less for women and 1,800 calories or less for men.

Reducing calories, however, means a reduction in the
amount of essential nutrients the body needs for optimal health.
Just to meet the daily RDI's for essential nutrients, you would
need to consume over 2,000 calories if you are a woman, and
3,000 if you are a man. Furthermore, when you take into
account all the factors that affect the nutrients in our food,
even eating well does not guarantee you are getting all the
nutrition you need. Instead of cutting calories to lose weight,
make a conscious effort to eat better. Avoid fast food, junk food,
and processed foods made with white flour and loaded with

sugar. Choose low-glycemic foods (see "The Low-Glycemic Diet" beginning on page 109).

The conservative *Journal of the American Medical Association (JAMA)* now recommends "all adults take one multivitamin daily." This recommendation was made after Harvard researchers reviewed thirty-year's worth of scientific studies and articles that focused on the relationship between vitamins and chronic disease conditions. The conclusions of this research were published by *JAMA* in 2002, after which Annette Dickinson, PhD, of the Council for Responsible Nutrition, commented, "There is no question that the amount of scientific evidence in favor of the consistent use of vitamins, particularly multivitamins, is formidable and must be taken seriously." Unfortunately, many physicians do not take this issue seriously. They leave their patients potentially uninformed about the many health benefits a sensible nutritional supplement program can provide.

INDUSTRY DIFFERENCES

Perhaps the biggest reason so many people are unaware of the complete range of available nutritional healthcare choices is due to advertising dollars. Marketing money spent by manufacturers of nutritional supplements is only a fraction of the amount spent each year by pharmaceutical companies on their drugs. This has been particularly obvious since 1998, when the Food and Drug Administration (FDA) lifted a moratorium that had prevented the pharmaceutical industry from engaging in direct-to-consumer advertising. Since that time, pharmaceutical companies have devoted the lion's share of their annual advertising budget's product promotion on television and radio, as well as in newspapers, consumer magazines, and on Internet websites.

As a result of such aggressive marketing practices, consumer demand for pharmaceutical drugs, particularly newly approved products, which are typically more expensive than older generic brands, has skyrocketed. In addition, as a result of the FDA's decision, drug companies are now allowed to run ads that urge consumers to ask their doctors about drugs they might not even need, often causing physicians to prescribe the drugs solely because their patients ask for them. Today, in part because of such advertising, Americans spend over $230 billion on pharmaceutical drugs annually. And that figure is growing by an average of 12 percent a year, making the cost of medications the fastest growing area of our nation's healthcare bill.

According to Pharmaceutical Research and Manufacturers of America (PhRMA)—a lobbyist group for the pharmaceutical industry based in Washington, DC—in 2003 alone, drug companies spent $25.3 billion on "drug promotional activities." Of that amount, approximately $3.3 billion was spent on direct-to-consumer advertising; $5.7 billion was spent on ads in medical journals and promotional material for doctors' offices and hospitals; and more than $16 billion was spent in the form of free samples of primarily newly approved drugs to physicians, who are encouraged to make them available to their patients. This is a clever way in which the drug companies improve the likelihood that patients will ask for these drugs.

The amount of money Americans spend each year on natural, alternative medical treatments is estimated at $27 billion (nearly all of which is paid out-of-pocket by consumers). Compare that to the $230 billion dollars spent annually on pharmaceuticals, and one has to believe that this amount is a reflection of the industry's staggering advertising budget. Imagine how much more likely consumers would be to try supplements and other natural products if the alternative health industry was in a position to give away $16 billion worth of its products every year. Obviously, this is not going to happen. It is, however, important for consumers to realize the disparity that exists between these industries in achieving public awareness for their products.

All Claims Are Not Created Equal

Another factor that must be considered when assessing the difference between pharmaceutical companies and manufacturers of nutritional supplements is the legitimacy of their product claims. And there is *much* to be considered.

The Natural Origins of Pharmaceuticals

Approximately 40 percent of all pharmaceutical drugs are derived from medicinal plants or herbs. In fact, the word "drug" is a derivative of the Dutch word *drogge,* which means "to dry." Prior to modern drug preparation methods, both physicians and traditional native healers commonly dried plants before using them medicinally.

Aspirin, one of the most common drugs, is derived from willow bark, an herb that is rich in salicin. The ancient Romans first recorded the use of willow bark as a treatment for fever; the Greek physician Hippocrates— "The Father of Medicine"—also prescribed it for the relief of pain. For centuries, Native American healers of the Great Plains states have used willow bark for its analgesic (pain-relieving) properties. Based on this herb's traditional use, nineteenth-century German chemists were able to synthesize its active ingredient, which led to the development of aspirin. Although aspirin and traditional willow bark preparations are both effective in reducing pain and fever, there is a major difference between them. Aspirin, considered one of the safest of all pharmaceutical drugs, can thin the stomach lining and cause internal bleeding. This adverse side effect is implicated in the deaths of anywhere from hundreds to thousands of Americans each year.

Critics of the nutritional supplement industry often charge that its product claims are unsubstantiated and the products themselves are potentially dangerous. While it's true that some supplement companies have made misleading product claims, this is not typical of reputable companies that have a legitimate spot in the marketplace.

As for the issue of safety, whenever there have been reported instances (although rare) of adverse effects caused by the use of certain nutritional supplements, the overall practices of the supplement industry as a whole were invariably called into question. The FDA usually moved into action quickly to remove such products from the marketplace. For example, when weight-loss supplements containing ephedra were implicated in 153 deaths, they were banned from consumer use. However, in each of these cases,

Other conventional medicines that are derived from medicinal plants include the drug AZT, used in the treatment of AIDS; digitalis, a cardiac stimulant; quinine, used to treat malaria; morphine, a pain killer; and Taxol, commonly prescribed for treating cancer. Vinblastine and vincristine, common drugs for the treatment of acute lymphocytic leukemia, also have their origins in medicinal plants.

There is an undeniable link between natural medicinal treatments and modern medicine. A greater awareness of this connection would help create a broader acceptance of the role nutritional supplements can play in overall preventive and therapeutic healthcare regimens. It would also help speed public knowledge and understanding of the value of such supplements.

It is interesting to note that the majority of natural supplements have been available for decades, centuries, and even (in the case of herbs) millennia. And yet, many of these products are only now coming to be commonly accepted by conventional physicians and the public at large. Creating public awareness of new natural supplements is even more difficult. Compared to pharmaceutical drugs, which typically enjoy the marketing push of corporate giants, breakthrough natural products are at a disadvantage when it comes to visibility in the marketplace.

the ephedra had not been taken according to labeling instructions. (Further information on ephedra's alleged role in these deaths is discussed later in this section.)

A federal judge later ruled that the FDA went too far in its action against ephedra, and rescinded the ban on products containing 10 milligrams or less. It's also important to point out that when the FDA enacted this ban, it did so selectively. It ruled that the use of ephedra by practitioners of acupuncture and traditional Chinese medicine for treating respiratory conditions (its use for centuries in China) was still allowed. Most interesting, the FDA took no action against common over-the-counter drugs that contained pseudoephedrine—a synthetic version of ephedra that is often found in decongestants and other nonprescription drugs.

As health practitioners who have dedicated our lives to researching the best possible healthcare options for our patients, we strongly agree with any FDA decision to remove any substance from the marketplace that causes serious adverse reactions. We also strongly support the FDA's stance against inaccurate or exaggerated claims relating to health products. Our concerns with the FDA's implementation of its regulatory responsibilities, however, is in the seemingly selective way it determines and implements its decisions regarding post-market surveillance of drugs and supplements after their release to the consumer. The FDA appears to lack balance, manpower, and focus in policing its regulatory obligations. Simply put, the FDA appears to place much greater focus on nutritional supplements than it does on prescription drugs. Why do we feel this way? Read on.

According to a 2004 study conducted by the Institute for Evidence-Based Medicine in Germany, 94 percent of the medical claims and information contained in promotional literature sent to doctors by pharmaceutical companies has no basis in scientific fact. In other words, the majority of claims and information are inaccurate and misleading. What follows are just a few of the Institute's findings:

- Medical guidelines from scientific groups are frequently misquoted.

- Side effects of drugs are minimized.

- Groups of patients are wrongly defined due to improper or misdiagnoses.

- Study results that adversely reflect the tested drugs are often suppressed.

- Treatment effects and benefits are exaggerated.

- Risks are manipulated to enhance the perception of safety.

- Many of the positively touted effects of drugs are drawn from animal (not human) studies, although the drugs are intended for human use.

Were a similar level of inaccuracy to be contained in promotional literature supplied by the manufacturers of natural supplements, the FDA would be likely to take immediate and strict actions against it. When it comes to the pharmaceutical industry, however, the FDA typically does little more than issue warnings without any further regulation.

One of the most serious issues we have with the FDA is its lack of speed in identifying post-market safety problems with pharmaceutical drugs and then following with regulating remedies. According to published reports in the *Journal of the American Medical Association, New England Journal of Medicine,* and other medical journals, each year, properly prescribed FDA-approved pharmaceutical drugs are implicated in the deaths of over 100,000 Americans, the hospitalization of at least 2 million others, and the harmful (although less-serious) side effects of approximately 20 million more.

By comparison, the total number of reported adverse reactions caused by "use as directed" nutritional supplements each year is infinitesimal. For example, the 153 deaths allegedly caused by ephedra supplements (discussed earlier) occurred over a number of years. In addition, most of these cases were unconfirmed. Moreover, scientific studies on ephedrine-caffeine combinations for weight loss in very overweight and obese adults and adolescents who are otherwise healthy, all concluded that they are safe and effective when used as directed. Furthermore, in many of these cases, the supplements were not taken in the prudent suggested doses; rather they were ingested in greater amounts than recommended, offering another possible cause of the extreme reaction.

Regarding the scope of adverse reactions associated with supplement use, it's important to recognize that in the category of vitamin and minerals, not a single death has been reported in peer review literature when they have been taken as properly prescribed (within their recommended preventive or therapeutic dosage range). It seems prudent, therefore, that the FDA, along with congressional support, might better fulfill its mission to protect public safety by properly directing its limited resources on regulating the drug industry and the supplement industry equally.

This focus should include not only due diligence in the drug-approval process and the regulation of supplements according to the Dietary Supplement Health and Education Act (DSHEA) guidelines, but also, and just as important, the implementation of quality post-market surveillance programs for both.

The COX-2 Inhibitor Problem

One of the most glaring and disturbing examples of the FDA's need to refine its current post-market surveillance and regulation of the pharmaceutical industry involves a group of drugs known as COX-2 inhibitors. Sold under the popular brand names Vioxx, Bextra, and Celebrex, these drugs have been prescribed for the treatment of arthritis and the management of acute pain.

Vioxx, the most popular of these drugs, which was approved by the FDA in 1999, was targeted as the cause of heart attack and stroke in over 139,000 consumers, beginning in 2001. Of those affected, at least 27,000 died. It was not until 2004, however, that drug company giant Merck, the manufacturer of Vioxx, voluntarily withdrew the drug from the marketplace—but not before Vioxx generated approximately $2.5 billion in revenues for the company.

Since then, information has surfaced indicating that Merck officials knew of the Vioxx's potential for causing heart attack and stroke, but kept this information from the FDA during its approval process of the drug. In fact, copies of Merck's internal files show that the company's officials knew about the drug's potential for causing these serious reactions in 1998, one year before the FDA approved Vioxx. Records also show that, in an effort to secure approval, Merck officials actively sought to prevent the FDA from discovering the drug's safety risks.

Based on this evidence, critics of Merck charged that the company is guilty of criminal behavior; currently a class action civil suit is being prepared against it. To date, however, the FDA has taken no action against Merck, despite the reaction of Dr. David Graham, associate director of the FDA's Office of Drug Safety. Dr. Graham called the FDA's original approval of Vioxx "The single greatest drug safety catastrophe in the history of this country or the history of this world." Furthermore, after Vioxx's life-threatening side effects became public in 2004, an FDA safety panel recommended that Vioxx and other COX-2 inhibitor drugs be allowed to return to the marketplace. There was one stipulation—the packaging had to contain a "black box" warning of the drug's implication in heart attack and stroke. (It was later revealed that more than half of the panel's eighteen members—all of whom voted in favor of the black box warnings instead of censuring the drug companies in any way—had current or former financial ties to the manufacturers of the assessed drugs.)

As a class of drugs, COX-2 inhibitors were among the most heavily promoted in the history of the pharmaceutical industry, resulting in their rapid popularity among patients and physicians alike. According to a report by the *San Francisco Chronicle*, in 2003 alone, the manufacturers of Vioxx, Bextra, and Celebrex "spent more than $1.5 billion to promote the drugs through television spots, print ads and pitches to doctors." In that year, Merck alone spent $499.8 million promoting Vioxx to doctors, and another $78 million touting the drug's benefits in direct-to-consumer ad campaigns. Merck's advertising efforts resulted in the sale of 19.9 million prescriptions of Vioxx that year, generating $1.8 billion in revenues for the company.

This is just one example of the imbalance between nutritional supplement companies and pharmaceutical manufacturers regarding the allocation of resources. If a nutritional supplement company was responsible for the same type of behavior exhibited by Merck in this example, and its supplement went on to cause the deaths of 27,000 people, the FDA would have acted much differently. At the very least, the nutrient company would be hit with heavy fines and its product would be banned from the marketplace. More than likely, criminal charges would also be brought against the company, followed by lengthy jail sentences for those company officials who knowingly hid the truth about their product.

Other Considerations

In addition to the major differences between the pharmaceutical and natural product industries just presented, other factors further highlight the drug industry's advantageous position.

Drug companies fund their own research. They pay for the toxicology, safety, and efficacy studies—everything that is related to the approval of their drug. Much of this data isn't published, which means an independent reviewer (outside the company) never critically reviewed it. To prevent any conflict of interest, the FDA should require independent research for these studies. (It does require independent review panels, but not independent research.) On the other hand, when a dietary supplement company funds research and submits it to a medical or scientific journal, independent reviewers who are not associated with the company evaluate the data. Acceptance for publication means it has passed the peer review process. Skeptics, however, may indicate that since the supplement company funded the study, the results are suspect. However, we believe reasonable review methodologies would certainly safeguard against possible conflicts. Furthermore, ethical nutritional companies would welcome processes that reward and protect excellence in safety and effectiveness.

There is yet another example of how drug companies have an advantage over natural product manufacturers—health insurance. The disturbing truth is that insurance companies will dole out exorbitant amounts for prescription drugs, but offer very little if anything in the way of co-payment opportunities for natural supplements or other preventive health measures. While this situation is gradually changing, the insurance coverage gap between drugs, medical procedures, and natural supplements is too large for the best interests of consumers.

The material presented in this chapter thus far has pointed out the clear differences in the way the FDA oversees the pharmaceutical industry and the manufacturers of nutritional supplements. It has also shown the amazing disparity in the amount of money spent by these two industries in creating public demand for their products. Through all of this information, it's easy to see why nutritional supplements typically take far longer to gain public awareness than it does for pharmaceutical drugs. Keeping this fact in mind, it's time to take a look at one man's vision and efforts, which have focused on ensuring that those who suffer from arthritis and other joint pain conditions become aware of a safe, natural, and effective alternative to potentially dangerous arthritis medications.

THE EARTH'S UNIQUE TREASURES

More than four billion years ago, as the earth's surface cooled, the geography of the planet emerged, giving way to the formation of mountains and valleys, rivers and lakes, and eventually oceans and seas. Grand land masses rose and fell, shifted and moved. Tremendous pressures beneath the earth's crust, along with the heat of escaping molten rock, and the constant forces of weathering and erosion, caused the redistribution of minerals—nature's true building blocks—throughout the land. Living organisms arose from the earth—first simple, and then more complex. And even as life spread through the planet, the forces of nature continued to create unique blends of the earth's elements. It is within this context that the following story begins.

An Amazing Discovery

Over a million years had passed since geo- and hydrothermal forces combined to create the unique mineral deposit found in the soil of the high Sierra Mountains. It was, however, the lure of gold that drew thousands of prospectors there over the past 150 years. In the 1970s, as one of those prospectors traveled through the mountains in search of golden treasure, he noticed that the soil sparkled when it was exposed to sunlight. He had come upon the rich Sierra mineral deposit.

After careful examination, the prospector soon realized that the soil did not contain a measurable amount of gold, yet he intuitively felt the area was worth mining. He laid claim to the area and set about looking for his treasure. During his early explorations, he noticed that the land contained a significant amount of natural clay. The prospector knew that natural clay had been prized for centuries by indigenous peoples, including Native Americans, who used it for a variety of health purposes and healing properties. When one of his dogs became lame in one paw, he decided to test the folklore remedy. He began adding some of the mineral-rich clay powder to the dog's food. After a few days, the dog exhibited noticeable improvements in both its ability to move around and its overall health. After that, whenever the prospector's other animals showed signs of pain or difficulty when walking, he began giving them the powder, which had the same positive effects.

Prospecting is not an easy job. It involves physical exertion, exposure to extreme temperatures, bumps and bruises, and the occasional accident. The miner's body pays a price—and the prospector in our story was no exception. He suffered from a host of bodily aches and pains, some caused by the physical aspects of his job, others from arthritis and rheumatism. Without the aid of a local doctor or pharmacy, he made do with what he had. After seeing the positive results the clay had on his dog, the prospector reckoned it might be helpful for his own condition. He began ingesting some of the clay powder himself, and the pain he had lived with for years vanished. The prospector had unexpectedly rediscovered what the local Native Americans had known for many years—nature truly provides.

Some time later, the prospector met a businessman, who had come to this remote area of the Sierra Mountains to pursue his passion for fly-fishing. As the two men got to know each other, the prospector eventually related his discovery of the mineral deposit and the healing effects it appeared to have on him and his animals. The businessman reasoned that the soil might be more of a treasure than the prospector had ever thought possible. The two men decided to form a partnership, and they acquired the mining rights to the Sierra deposit.

Shortly after the businessman had financed the initial mining of the deposit, he began giving samples of the mineral powder to people he knew. Together, they began ingesting small amounts each day with water. Soon, they began to notice improvements in their health, with the reduction of joint pain the most common and significant benefit. Although the businessman brought in other investors, he did not have enough funding to commercialize the find. However, he and his friends and associates continued to make the mineral soil part of their daily health regimen.

In 2001, an associate of the businessman decided to seek business counsel and investment advice from Peter Bentley, with whom he had previously been involved in another joint venture. Bentley—the distinguished Chairman of the Board of the multibillion-dollar Canfor Corporation (Canada's leading integrated forest products company), as well as the Chairman of Canadian Forest Products, Ltd. (Canfor's principal subsidiary)—was indeed well qualified to provide valuable advice for the group. Among his many other business accomplishments, Bentley also served for many years as a director of the Bank of Montreal and Shell Canada, Ltd., and he is the current chancellor of the University of Northern British Columbia.

At the time of the initial meeting, Bentley was seventy years old and had been suffering with arthritic hands for a few years. The increasing joint pain was limiting his ability to participate in a number of activities, including his beloved game of golf. He had exhausted many of the common conventional arthritis treatments, including all of the pharmaceutical drugs. None provided lasting relief.

The businessman entered Bentley's office with samples of the mineral-rich powder and told Bentley that he and his partners believed that it was the solution for arthritis. Because modern medicine had failed Bentley in relieving his own arthritis symptoms, he was naturally very skeptical, and had no difficulty in saying so. But the businessman persisted, sharing with Bentley the results he and others had experienced shortly after ingesting the powder.

Although he remained skeptical, Bentley's interest was piqued. When he learned all he had to do was add a teaspoon of the powder to a glass of water and drink it every morning, he agreed to give it a try. Within days, Bentley experienced significant improvement in his hands. He was intrigued. He was also delighted, and immediately ordered a large supply of the powder, which he continued taking daily.

Bentley began handing out samples to his friends who also suffered from arthritis and other joint-pain conditions. Before long, they too were reporting that their arthritis pains and related symptoms were gone or significantly improved. One of his friends, who had been scheduled for shoulder surgery that summer, began taking the powder in April. Within a few weeks, he was totally pain free and had canceled the surgery. Another friend, who was also about to undergo surgery because of the excruciating pain in both knees, started taking the powder. The results he experienced were nothing short of amazing. Within just three days, the pain in his knees was gone.

This is just a sampling of the positive feedback Bentley began receiving from the people with whom he had shared the mineral powder. In nearly every instance, encouraging results began to occur within a matter of days. (For the detailed account of his friend and 1964 US Open Golf Champion, Ken Venturi, see "Back in the Swing" on page 54.)

Bentley had no idea how the powder worked. All he knew was that it did. As the samples Bentley gave out started to encompass a growing circle of people, he received another surprise. Users began reporting that the powder was helping more than their arthritis. In many cases, it had also resolved or significantly relieved symptoms of other chronic health conditions, including osteoporosis and Crohn's disease—a condition characterized by chronic inflammation of the gastrointestinal tract, and resulting in such symptoms as abdominal pain, chronic diarrhea, fever, headaches, and malabsorption.

Although Bentley did not understand how the soil worked, he was completely convinced of its healing properties. He recognized it as a treatment that could potentially benefit millions of people. After becoming an initial investor in the businessman's mining venture, Bentley acquired rights to the mineral deposit. On Christmas Eve of 2003, he and his son Michael formed the company Sierra Mountain Minerals, Inc. They called the mineral compound *SierraSil,* named for the Sierra Mountains, where it is found, and the primary minerals it contains called *silicates.*

Both Bentleys—father and son—recognized the potential benefits that the SierraSil mineral complex could offer those who suffered with arthritis. Having finally found a treatment that actually worked to end his own crippling arthritis pain, Peter especially believed in the product. It became his personal mission to share this "mineral miracle" with others. Being an astute businessman, however, he realized that bringing such a product to market would not be easy. He knew that he had to overcome the obstacles that stood in the way of all new and innovative natural health aids before they came to be accepted. His mission was one that required careful planning.

Although Bentley knew the SierraSil complex worked for him, as well as his friends and associates, he also realized that such reports were anecdotal and would certainly be dismissed by the conventional arthritis establishment. To respond to such objections, both Bentley and his son realized that they had to know the following information about SierraSil: 1) how safe it is for ongoing human consumption, 2) how it works, and 3) if scientific studies could verify the results that Bentley and many others had personally experienced.

Knowing this information about *any* new product requires a great deal of time and funding. For this reason, many nutritional supplement manufacturers rely solely on anecdotal reports when marketing their products. But the Bentleys knew that to be successful in their mission, the SierraSil powder had to undergo rigorous, extensive scientific studies. It was important to determine the nature of the powder's healing properties. Fortunately, the Bentley's were in a position to underwrite the costs of such studies, which will be discussed in Chapter 3.

More to the Story

In addition to underwriting the cost of the SierraSil research, the Bentleys wanted to find out if there was something about the deposit itself that had something to do with the powder's healing properties. So they hired Dr. Haydn Murray, one of the world's leading mineralogists, to evaluate the SierraSil mineral deposit.

After conducting a process called *x-ray diffraction analysis* to study the deposit, Dr. Murray stated, "In my more than fifty years of mineral research, I have never seen a combination of minerals like this before. The parent igneous rock material was altered by an underground hot water solution that resulted in a very unusual mineral suite." Clearly, there *is* something about the mineral

Back in the Swing

One of the biggest disappointments Peter Bentley experienced as his arthritis pain progressed was that it forced him to curtail golfing, a sport he passionately enjoyed. Within a week of taking the SierraSil on a daily basis, all of Bentley's arthritis pain disappeared. After living with the pain for years (in spite of trying every available treatment option), Bentley viewed his new pain-free state as miraculous. He was especially pleased that he was able to enjoy himself on the golf course again without any discomfort.

One of Bentley's close friends, Ken Venturi, became a professional golfer in 1956 and began competing on the PGA Tour. The most dramatic of his fourteen tour wins was the 1964 US Open. Later that year, the PGA named him Player of the Year, and *Sports Illustrated* honored him as Sportsman of the Year. Unfortunately, Venturi's tenure as a professional golfer proved to be short-lived. In 1965, he began to lose feeling in his hands and started dropping golf balls during rounds. He also developed pain, which was treated unsuccessfully with cortisone shots. Venturi was diagnosed with carpal tunnel syndrome.

Unwilling to give up his career or the game he loved, Venturi underwent surgery, after which he began playing professional tournaments again. Unfortunately, his level of play over the next three years was mediocre at best, forcing his retirement as a professional golfer in 1968. That same year, in order to stay close to the game, Venturi began a second career as lead golf analyst for CBS Sports, which continued for thirty-five years. He became the longest-running leading television analyst in the history of sports. During that time, however, Venturi's physical condition continued to deteriorate and he required further surgery on his hands. Eventually, he developed arthritis, which severely compounded his old injuries and surgical scars. Although he tried every known treatment to reverse his condition, nothing worked. His hopes of ever playing golf again, even socially, seemed to be over once and for all.

Everything changed when Bentley told Venturi about his own amazing recovery after taking the SierraSil powder. He encouraged Venturi to try it. To his astonishment, Venturi soon discovered that his own arthritis pain was lessening. Before long, he, too, was able to return to the golf course.

So impressed was Venturi by the miraculous change that occurred after taking the SierraSil, he submitted an official testimonial to the US House Subcommittee on Human Rights and Wellness, chaired by Congressman Dan Burton (R) of Indiana in 2004. In his testimony, Venturi stated, "SierraSil has helped me more than anything else I've ever tried. It's been amazing! This supplement has given me back my hand strength, and I have more flexibility than before. I'm finally able to play golf again, which I certainly haven't done in years. I'm back to hitting golf balls almost every day, and I've picked up distance again. The SierraSil is just incredible. I just feel great."

Venturi concluded his testimony by urging the members of the US House of Representatives to do whatever they could to ensure that dietary supplements, like the SierraSil mineral complex, as well as information about their health-enhancing benefits, are easily available.

deposit that makes the SierraSil compound unique and unlike any other mineral sampling in the world. Armed with this knowledge, the Bentleys were ready to proceed with the scientific studies.

CONCLUSION

With a clear understanding of what needed to be done—as well as the potential obstacles that lay in front of them—the Bentleys took on the daunting challenge of bringing a new natural product to market. This choice was not based solely on financial gain, for Peter Bentley had already achieved both commercial prominence and financial independence years before. The decision to move ahead was fueled by the desire to share a discovery that could offer a natural, effective means of relieving pain to millions of people with absolutely no adverse side effects.

The next chapter covers the extensive scientific testing and evaluation of SierraSil that the Bentleys required to meet their own uncompromising standards. This testing stage was designed to avoid the roadblocks that have stopped so many other natural products from gaining recognition.

CHAPTER 3

The Science Behind SierraSil

As you saw in Chapter 2, after trying every known treatment for his chronic arthritis pain, Peter Bentley experienced almost immediate relief when he began taking the SierraSil mineral complex. So impressed was he with the results, he offered it to many of his friends and associates who also suffered with joint pain from arthritis or other inflammatory conditions. They reported equally significant relief. Knowing the available treatments in the marketplace either didn't work or did so at the cost of increased health risks, Bentley felt compelled to get out the word on SierraSil. He wanted to share this important discovery with others so they, too, could experience joint pain relief.

Bentley realized, however, that before presenting this information to the public, he needed more than anecdotal evidence to back it up. Knowing how the compound had achieved its beneficial effects and whether it was safe for long-time use was key. Although this step required time and a substantial amount of money, Bentley knew it was crucial—and he was driven in his goal to help others who were suffering as he once did. After setting up Sierra Mountain Minerals, Inc., Bentley and his son underwrote the costs of the research and scientific studies on the SierraSil mineral complex. They had to be sure that it was safe and effective for long-term use as a natural health supplement. This chapter presents that research and its findings.

SAFETY FIRST

The first studies conducted on the SierraSil powder focused on its safety. Although it is certainly impressive for a nutritional supplement or medication to provide relief from joint pain, as SierraSil clearly does, it also has to be safe. Drugs like Vioxx and other COX-2 inhibitors may be effective for relieving arthritis pain, but they also dramatically increase the risk of heart attack and stroke. As discussed in the last chapter, Vioxx alone was reportedly responsible for the deaths of at least 27,000 people before Merck pulled it from the marketplace. There was also the case of the weight-loss supplements containing ephedra, which were implicated in 153 deaths. The point here is that it is vitally important to know that the supplement or medication you are taking is safe for long-term use.

In compliance with the Dietary Supplement Health and Education Act of 1994, the Bentleys financed a series of industry standard tests to determine the safety of the SierraSil powder. Commonly used to evaluate the safety of health products, foods, agricultural products, and pharmaceutical compounds for human use, these tests included the following: a 14-Day Acute Oral LD50 Toxicity study, a 90-Day Sub-Acute Oral Toxicity study, a Dissolution test, and an Ames test. This intense level of safety testing is seldom seen within the nutriceutical industry. The Bentleys, however, demanded it, and the results were impressive. SierraSil came through all of the tests with zero indication of toxicity. Let's take a closer look at each of the tests now.

Of all the safety tests SierraSil underwent, the 90-Day Sub-Acute Oral Toxicity test was possibly the most important due to its lengthy duration and high dosage amounts. During this test, lab animals were fed doses of SierraSil that ranged as high as the equivalent of thirty-five times the recommended daily dose for humans. This was done for a period of ninety days. It is important to note that the standard length for this test is twenty-eight days, but the Bentleys, in an effort to be even more thorough, instructed that the test last three times longer than the norm.

Throughout the test and for a twenty-eight day recovery period afterward, the test animals were monitored for health, dietary habits, and behavior. It was noted that they had all gained weight. At the end of the test, the animals were euthanized and their major organs were examined under a microscope. No abnormalities were observed. In addition, the animals' livers were analyzed for iron, aluminum, arsenic, and lead—the less-desirable minerals contained in SierraSil. No accumulation was found, as even the high-dose animals were found to have only background levels of these minerals. Because there was no buildup, the bioavailable amounts of these minerals in SierraSil have been assumed to be zero to low. (As discussed in Chapter 2, *bioavailability* refers to how much of a compound is available to the body's tissues and is taken up by those tissues.) The test concluded that SierraSil is safe at doses equivalent to thirty-five times the recommended daily clinical dose of 2 grams.

The term *bioaccessibility* is related to bioavailability. It refers to the quantity of a compound that is made accessible to the body during digestion. To determine its bioaccessibility, SierraSil entered a simulated gut environment through dissolution testing. The resulting liquid was tested for mineral content to determine—on a mineral-by-mineral basis—how much of each mineral left the solid phase and became accessible to the body for potential uptake. The test results were important because certain questionable minerals, such as lead, which are present in SierraSil in very low part-per-million quantities, did not leave the silicate mineral and, therefore, were not accessible to the body for potential uptake. Silicate minerals in general are known to bind minerals very tightly, and require strong acid or alkaline conditions outside those found in the human body to break the molecular bonds and release all of their component minerals.

The LD50 test has been used since 1927 to determine the potential toxicity of drugs and other medications, as well as nutritional supplements, food products, and environmental contaminants. Variations of this test are used for different applications to this day. The LD50 test is so named because it represents the amount of a substance that is a lethal dose (LD) to 50 percent or more of the animal subjects under test conditions.

For SierraSil, an Acute Oral LD50 test was employed. Labora-tory rats were fed the test substance at several dosage amounts for fourteen days to determine which dose, if any, caused significant mortality. Generally in an LD50 test, substances that kill half of the test population quickly are considered unsafe for human con-sumption. Substances that kill 50 percent of the test subjects after they have been given doses in much higher amounts than would be taken by humans may be considered safe or may require further testing. The lower the amount of a substance that is required to cause the death of 50 percent of the test animals, the higher its tox-icity. Conversely, the higher the amount that produces the same results, the safer it is for human consumption.

When SierraSil underwent the Acute Oral LD50 test, the results were a complete "failure" for producing toxic results. Even the test animals that were given dosages equivalent to seventy times high-er than the clinically recommended daily dose for humans showed absolutely no toxic effects. As a result, the test concluded that the Acute Oral LD50 for SierraSil is in excess of 2,000 milligrams per kilogram of body weight (greater than seventy times the recom-mended daily dose in humans). These results confirmed SierraSil's safety as a daily health supplement.

As another point of interest, during the Acute Oral LD50 test period, the rats actually exhibited improvements in their health, including healthy weight gain. Furthermore, once they stopped taking the SierraSil, follow-up testing (internal examination by sur-gery) showed no signs of illness. Instead, they maintained the healthy gains they had achieved during the study.

The last of SierraSil's initial safety tests was the Ames test. Named after its inventor, Bruce N. Ames, who developed it in 1974, the Ames test determines if a substance, once ingested by humans, acts as a carcinogen (cancer-causing agent). Specifically, it ascertains if the test substance can cause harmful mutagenic changes to cells and tissues. These changes or mutations are due to toxic substances called *mutagens*, which are capable of increas-ing the rate and frequency of cellular change.

During the Ames test, the substance being studied is put into contact with *Salmonella typhimurium*—a strain of Salmonella bacteria. This particular strain possesses a defective gene that causes the bacteria to mutate if it comes in contact with a test substance that is toxic or mutagenic. If mutation occurs, there is a strong likelihood that the test substance will act as a carcinogen when it is ingested and metabolized by the body. To ensure the most accurate results, animal liver enzymes are also added during this test; these enzymes mimic those that would be produced by the human liver once the test substance is consumed. The result of the Ames test made it clear that the SierraSil powder is not mutagenic.

The results of the all of these tests showed conclusively that SierraSil powder poses no risk of adverse health effects—even when taken consistently and in large amounts. It causes no harmful mutagenic changes or toxicity. In short, the scientific evidence clearly showed that the SierraSil compound is safe for human consumption on a daily, ongoing basis.

Once the safety of the SierraSil powder was established, the Bentleys turned their attention to discovering how and why it caused rapid and significant relief of arthritis pain.

HOW SIERRASIL WORKS

All medical treatments, whether natural or man-made, work in a specific manner to relieve or cure various disorders. Some products work by bolstering or restoring the body's immune system, while others enhance the ability of other systems in the body, such as the cardiovascular, circulatory, digestive, or respiratory systems. Still other products work by normalizing various body functions, or by reversing certain harmful effects, such as those caused by free radicals.

In order to discover how the SierraSil compound works, the Bentleys hired scientific researchers to conduct a "mechanism of action" (MOA) study. This type of study determines the effects of a tested substance on the body, as well as how it achieves those effects—this is considered the substance's mechanism of action. An MOA study seeks to determine which parts of the body the substance interacts with at the molecular level, and which of the body's biochemical and biological activities it affects or influences.

Mineral Toxicity
A Question of What You Absorb

When the Bentleys looked at the list of minerals that made up SierraSil's unique composition, their attention was drawn to the bottom lines of the report. In addition to the many beneficial macro- and trace minerals, the chemical analysis had detected minute traces of aluminum, arsenic, cadmium, iron, lead, and mercury. The Bentleys were concerned. Weren't these trace elements potentially harmful? The question of safety further heightened their need to carefully study any potential toxic risk, no matter how slight.

Their concerns were put to rest through a battery of tests that were conducted on the compound. Both the animal and human studies (detailed in this chapter) clearly revealed that SierraSil poses no danger of toxicity, even when consumed in dosages that are seventy times greater than the suggested daily allowance, and over long periods of time. You might wonder how this can be, given that SierraSil *does* contain the trace elements mentioned. The explanation is two-fold. First, the total percentage of the trace elements contained in the powder is extremely small in relation to its total composition. In fact, when compared with the same elements found in other naturally occurring substances, as well

To ensure that the MOA study was conducted according to the highest scientific standards, the Bentleys reached out to one of the world's leading research experts—Mark J.S. Miller, PhD, Professor of Cardiovascular Sciences and Pediatrics at New York State's Albany Medical College—to oversee the testing. Dr. Miller is also a grant recipient for conducting research for the National Institutes of Health (NIH).

To understand the details of the MOA study, which focused on SierraSil's effect on arthritis (specifically osteoarthritis), and the significance of its results, it is important to first understand what arthritis is and how it affects the body. Arthritis refers to inflammatory diseases that affect the joints, and whose overall symptoms include joint inflammation, pain, and stiffness. It is not a single disease, but many, with rheumatoid and osteoarthritis as the two major forms.

as many available commercial food products, SierraSil's amounts ranked very low on these lists. To see just how low, see the "Comparative Mineral Charts," beginning on page 141.

Second, these specific trace elements have zero to low bioavailability, which means they have little chance of being absorbed by the body. Rather, they pass through harmlessly until the body eventually eliminates them, the same way dietary fiber passes through largely undigested. This question of absorption is very important when exploring toxicity, because it is only when potentially harmful substances are absorbed that they are able to cause the body harm.

An analysis of the element composition contained in the SierraSil product revealed that this natural mineral complex contains a perfect balance of elements that work together in the body therapeutically—without producing adverse side effects. Moreover, the primary health-enhancing minerals contained in SierraSil prevent any potentially harmful elements from being absorbed. For example, calcium blocks the absorption of lead; zinc blocks the absorption of cadmium. Both calcium and zinc are among the many beneficial minerals contained in SierraSil. This perfect balance of elements ensures the compound's benefits without concern of negative side effects.

Rheumatoid arthritis is considered an autoimmune disease in which the body's immune system mistakenly attacks the tissues of the musculoskeletal system during the primary phase of the disease process. Eventually, during the second phase of the advancing disease, major organs become critical targets as well. However, during the primary phase, this "out-of-control" attack causes degeneration of the cartilage and joints, most often of the hands, wrists, feet, ankles, and knees.

Recent research provides evidence that various (chronic) nutrient deficiencies (i.e. minerals and glyconutrients) cause an interruption of healthy tissue production. This impairs the body's ability to form the correct three-dimensional structure of "glycoproteins," which also require certain minerals. Glycoproteins include collagen and immune complexes (like IgG), which are responsible for identifying if a substance is friend or foe to the body. In the case of rheumatoid arthritis, if the IgG detects that the collagen is "imperfect" it identifies it as a "foe" and signals an increase in immune system attack on the "enemy" collagen.

At the onset of this condition, the synovial cell membrane, which surrounds the joints and keeps them lubricated, becomes inflamed for the reasons just cited. This triggers the inflamed synovial cells to also produce oxidizing agents, which contribute to the synovial membrane's attack by the immune system. This, in turn, contributes to the breakdown of the cartilage surrounding the joints, leading to joint pain, stiffness, and eventual calcification.

Osteoarthritis, by contrast, is considered a degenerative disease in which the cartilage covering the ends of bones deteriorates. Most commonly caused by the wear and tear of aging, osteoarthritis can also be the result of injury or the abnormal development of the components of cartilage, such as collagen. With osteoarthritis, the normally smooth surface of the cartilage eventually becomes rough and pitted, interfering with joint mobility and its ability to properly absorb impact. The occurrence of any of these causative factors leads to stimulation of the *chondrocyte cells,* which are contained within the cartilage. When activated, chondrocytes cause the cartilage to deteriorate, a process known as *catabolism*. The end result is crippling joint pain and impaired movement.

To determine SierraSil's mechanism of action, Dr. Miller and his colleagues acquired slices of human cartilage taken from the knees of patients with severe osteoarthritis who were undergoing knee replacement surgery. During the study, the cartilage samples were combined with interleukin-1beta (IL-1B), a substance that is the primary initiator of the cartilage destruction associated with both osteoarthritis and rheumatoid arthritis. As IL-1B comes in contact with cartilage, it activates the chondrocyte cells. As mentioned earlier, when activated, chondrocytes start to destroy the cartilage itself, as well as promote the generalized inflammation that is characteristic of arthritis. Dr. Miller chose this approach for his research for two reasons: It was able to be well-controlled, and it accurately mirrored the inflammatory arthritic processes that occur in the human body.

While the cartilage test samples were being prepared with IL-1B to stimulate chondrocyte cells, the SierraSil compound was separated into three batches—one batch was subjected to a neutral wash, another to an alkaline wash, and the third to an acid wash. Three additional batches of the SierraSil compound were prepared in combination with Vincaria (an anti-inflammatory extract of the herb cat's claw). These batches were also subjected to neutral, alkaline, and acid washes. Each batch was then brought into contact with the prepared cartilage samples. The evaluation was based on two criteria—one involved the amount of nitric oxide produced by the chondrocytes, a sign of cartilage breakdown; the other involved how much glycosaminoglycan (GAG), a substance that breaks off from cartilage as it degenerates, was released.

During their evaluation, Dr. Miller and his colleagues found that neither the neutral nor the alkaline-washed plain SierraSil samples (without Vincaria) produced a significant reduction in the release of either nitric oxide or GAG. However, in the batches that also contained Vincaria, the release of both nitric oxide and GAG were reduced. Even more impressive, both of the acid-washed SierraSil samples—with and without Vincaria—exhibited the ability to dramatically reduce the production of both nitric oxide and GAG. Moreover, when they were introduced to the prepared cartilage samples, the reduction occurred rapidly. Because the stomach has an acidic environment, the acid-washed SierraSil samples closely reflected the compound's passage through the stomach when taken as a supplement. Let's further examine what these test results mean to anyone suffering from arthritic pain and chronic inflammation.

As discussed earlier, although the two major forms of arthritis may result from different factors, they both exhibit degeneration of the cartilage matrix due to chronic inflammation. This inflammation is caused by IL-1B, among other factors. As this inflammation process occurs, both nitric oxide and glycosaminoglycan (GAG) are also produced, leading to further ongoing cartilage and joint degeneration. Therefore, the key to supporting the stabilization, reversal, and/or prevention of arthritis lies in halting this degeneration process.

Dr. Miller's research showed that this is precisely what the SierraSil mineral compound does; moreover, it begins to do so almost immediately. But his study's most important discovery was that the SierraSil powder *actually suppresses the gene expression that is responsible for unhealthy inflammation in the body.* Commenting on the results, Dr. Miller said, "The mechanism of action study showed that SierraSil prevented the loss of cartilage structure and inflammation." Although the MOA study was specifically tailored to research how the SierraSil minerals affected osteoarthritis, Dr. Miller added, "I think that you can interpret that SierraSil will work for a wide range of joint conditions, as well as other chronic inflammation states."

To summarize, the MOA study revealed that the SierraSil minerals work to directly inhibit the primary inflammatory cascade that causes osteoarthritis. Based on the study's findings, we agree with Dr. Miller's assessment that the SierraSil compound is also an effective treatment for rheumatoid arthritis and other types of joint problems, since chronic inflammation is their primary cause. Inhibiting inflammation in the manner that the SierraSil minerals do is something that, to our knowledge, no other nutritional supplement is capable of doing.

Comparing SierraSil Support to Other Arthritis Treatments

Prior to the discovery of the SierraSil mineral compound, the treatment options available for rheumatoid arthritis, osteoarthritis, and other joint diseases were pharmaceutical drugs, nutritional supplements such as glucosamine and chondroitin, and, in severe cases of osteoarthritis, surgery and joint replacement.

Analgesics (painkillers) are the common drug treatment for arthritis and other joint diseases. They include acetaminophen (Tylenol, Datril); and nonsteroidal anti-inflammatory drugs (NSAIDs), such as aspirin, ibuprofen, ketoprofen, naproxen sodium, and COX-2 inhibitors (Bextra, Celebrex, and Vioxx). All of these drugs are prescribed for both osteoarthritis and rheumatoid arthritis. Those with rheumatoid arthritis may also use corticosteroids, such as prednisone; so-called "slow-acting drugs," such as gold compounds, penicillamine, and sufasalazine; and tissue necrosis factor (TNF)-alpha blocking agents, such as humira.

New Research Reveals Further Health Risks of Common Pain-Relief Drugs

In the United States, two of the most commonly used drugs are acetaminophen (Tylenol, Datril) and ibuprofen (Advil, Motrin, Nuprin), which, along with aspirin, are used by an estimated 32 million Americans to help relieve the pain of arthritis and other inflammatory conditions. Recent research, however, suggests that both acetaminophen and ibuprofen can greatly increase the risk of developing high blood pressure—a major contributor to both heart disease and stroke—in women.

According to the results of a recent study conducted by researchers at Brigham and Women's Hospital and published in the medical journal *Hypertension,* women with arthritis who regularly use acetaminophen or ibuprofen have up to double the risk of developing high blood pressure compared to women with arthritis who use aspirin. (The researchers did, however, caution against switching to aspirin, which increases the risk of gastrointestinal bleeding.) Specifically, the study involved 1,903 women between fifty-one and seventy-seven years of age, and 3,220 women between the ages of thirty-four and fifty-three. None of the subjects had high blood pressure before the study began.

The researchers found that women in the older age group who took the 500 milligrams of acetaminophen (the equivalent of one extra-strength nonprescription tablet) each day were 93 percent more likely to develop high blood pressure than women who did not use the drug. In the younger age group, the risk of high blood pressure when using the same dosage increased to 99 percent.

Among the women in the older age group who used at least 400 milligrams of ibuprofen (the equivalent of two nonprescription tablets) per day, the risk of developing high blood pressure increased by 78 percent. Among the younger women, the risk increased to 60 percent. According to the *Los Angeles Times,* which reported on this study, "Although the researchers do not recommend that most women stop using pain relievers, they suggest alternatives in some cases."

None of the drug types just mentioned targets or resolves the causes of arthritis; they simply relieve the symptoms. And all of these drugs can cause serious, potentially fatal side effects. We have already discussed the tens of thousands of deaths due to heart attack and stroke that have been attributed to Vioxx. All told, according to Dr. David Graham, associate director in the FDA's Office of Drug Safety, "A staggering 88,000 to 139,000 Americans have suffered heart attacks or strokes as a result of taking Vioxx." Similarly disturbing statistics have been attributed to Bextra and Celebrex. Furthermore, COX-2 inhibitors are implicated in other dangerous side effects, including kidney problems and serious liver problems, such as hepatitis, jaundice, and even complete liver failure.

Even the NSAID aspirin (the so-called "safe" drug) is responsible for the deaths of anywhere from hundreds to thousands of Americans each year due to internal stomach bleeding. As a class, NSAIDs are responsible for more than 107,000 hospitalizations and over 16,000 deaths in the United States each year. That's more deaths than from AIDS. NSAIDs can also cause elevated blood pressure, serious kidney problems, and gastrointestinal conditions, such as stomach ulcers. When taken long-term, some NSAIDs can actually destroy cartilage.

According to the *Merck Manual,* a primary medical reference text, corticosteroids such as prednisone can cause "numerous side effects throughout the body." And harmful side effects among the slow-acting arthritis drugs, such as sulfasalazine, include itchy skin and/or rashes; kidney, liver, and stomach problems; blood cell disorders; suppressed blood cell production in the bone marrow; and muscle disease. Although all of these drugs can improve arthritis symptoms, based on all of their potential health threats, we strongly discourage their use.

Since the 1990s, increasing numbers of arthritis sufferers have turned to natural alternatives to help relieve their symptoms, with the supplements glucosamine and chondroitin as the most popular. Both of these nutrients are effective in relieving arthritis pain, and, unlike arthritis drugs, they are safe for long-term use. However, typically the relief they provide does not begin to take effect until after two or three months of continual use. This is one of the reasons we find the SierraSil mineral complex, which reportedly shows significant improvements in two weeks or less, superior to both glucosamine and chondroitin. In fact, as seen in the MOA study, SierraSil's protective effects occurred within only a few hours.

There is an even more important reason that we feel the SierraSil mineral complex (also referred to by its research code as SM317) is superior to other nutritional supplements. Although supplements, including glucosamine and chondroitin, are much safer than arthritis medications and can provide pain relief over time, like pharmaceutical drugs, they do not address the causes of arthritis. The SierraSil minerals do. According to Dr. Miller:

> The real key when it comes to effectively treating both rheumatoid and osteoarthritis is cartilage. The function of cartilage is to facilitate joint movement by providing a smooth surface between the joints. In a sense, cartilage can be likened to a Teflon coating between the bones. In both forms of arthritis, cartilage becomes degraded.
>
> If you think of cartilage as a brick wall, then this process of degradation and degeneration would be similar to bricks crumbling and collapsing from that wall. Keeping with this analogy, glucosamine and chondroitin are the equivalent of bricks for this wall. When you supplement with glucosamine and chondroitin, you are really just ingesting more bricks with the hope that they are going to be added to the cartilage in an orderly manner to rebuild the wall that has been destroyed. However, if you go to any building site and you order a ton of bricks, what you actually get is a pile of bricks. You don't get the wall.
>
> To effectively treat and reverse arthritis you need to regulate the process of actually replacing the bricks that have fallen from the wall while at the same time preventing, or at least limiting, any further destruction of the wall from occurring. That is not something that either glucosamine or chondroitin can do. When you supplement with them, you are simply ordering more bricks. Neither glucosamine nor chondroitin address the destructive process that is involved in arthritis, which continues unabated due to chronic inflammation.
>
> What happens during chronic inflammation is that various genes in the body that influence inflammation are turned on inappropriately. In a state of health, these genes turn on when inflammation is appropriate, such as for the repair of wounds

or injuries or to deal with invading pathogens such as bacteria and viruses, and then turn off when their tasks are completed. With chronic inflammation, however, the genes remain turned on permanently, leading to degeneration of cartilage.

The reason that the SierraSil minerals work so well for arthritis and other inflammatory conditions is because they actually negate this inflammatory process, rather than simply attempting to repair the cartilage wall while inflammation continues unabated. This is what distinguishes the SierraSil minerals from glucosamine, chondroitin, and other nutritional supplements. The SierraSil minerals actually reduce the inflammation, while these other supplements don't have any effect on the inflammation at all. They simply replace bits of cartilage that are lost as a result of inflammation, fighting against a tide of destruction, whereas the SierraSil minerals are actually halting the destructive process by blocking the inflammation.

Returning to our analogy of cartilage being like a brick wall, the SierraSil minerals actually stop the destruction of the wall, while, at the same time, activating the body's natural repair processes to replace the bricks that have crumbled or fallen from the wall. Unless you are able to stop the inflammatory process, these repair processes can't be activated and, therefore, can't do their jobs because the inflammatory process directly switches off the genes that are involved in repair. When you take the SierraSil minerals, you block the inflammation and enable the repair processes to do what they have to do in terms of joint repair and remodeling.

Clearly, it is better to address the cause of a disease or illness, than it is to simply treat its symptoms. The research of Dr. Miller and his colleagues showed that this is precisely what the SierraSil minerals do with regard to the underlying mechanisms that cause arthritis and various other joint disorders. Dr. Miller's study, establishing how the SierraSil minerals work, was published in the *Journal of the American Nutrition Association (JANA)* in 2004.

Once the researchers understood SierraSil's mechanism of action, the Bentleys continued their scientific investigation by underwriting a double-blind human clinical study. The purpose of this study was to determine if the results that Peter Bentley and his friends had experienced after taking the SierraSil minerals were consistent among other arthritis sufferers.

HUMAN TRIALS CONFIRM THAT SIERRASIL WORKS

Soon after the MOA study was complete, Dr. Miller conducted an initial pilot study on humans, which showed that the SierraSil minerals improved joint flexibility and overall quality of life in the study participants. Based on these positive results, Dr. Miller

The Healing Properties of Cat's Claw

Also known as *una de gato,* cat's claw is a healing herb that is indigenous to the Amazon rainforest and other tropical areas of Latin America. It is a large, woody vine and with thorns that resemble a cat's claws, hence its name. According to Leslie Taylor, ND, a leading expert in herbal medicine and author of *The Healing Power of Rainforest Herbs,* cat's claw has been used for at least 2,000 years by traditional native healers throughout Central and South America, especially in Peru. There, the Ashaninka Indian tribe has used it as a primary treatment for a variety of disease conditions, including arthritis, rheumatism, and bone pain, as well as a means of controlling inflammation. Ashaninka healers also use cat's claw to help reverse inflammation of the urinary tract, cleanse the kidneys, treat gastric ulcers, cleanse and heal deep wounds, and aid in the recovery from childbirth.

Since the early 1970s, researchers from around the world have studied the healing properties of cat's claw. In addition to reducing inflammation, it has been scientifically shown to stimulate immune function, enhance cell health, protect against free radical damage, detoxify the gastrointestinal tract, protect against gastrointestinal disorders, and destroy both cancer and leukemia cells. Cat's claw has also been shown to cleanse the blood, reduce high blood pressure and cholesterol levels, kill viruses, and relieve pain.

Vincaria is an extract of cat's claw. In the mechanism of action study conducted under the supervision of Dr. Mark J.S. Miller (see page 61), the addition of Vincaria to the SierraSil minerals enhanced their ability to literally turn off the underlying causes of cartilage degeneration.

devised and conducted a double-blind placebo-controlled study involving 107 osteoarthritis patients. The extensive scope of this study went far beyond the efforts of most manufacturers of nutritional supplements when affirming the benefits and safety of their products. The Bentleys and Dr. Miller felt, however, that such a test was critical to establish the effectiveness and safety of the SierraSil minerals.

When devising the study, Dr. Miller developed a protocol that was intended to enable comparisons of the results experienced by the test subjects who used the SierraSil minerals, with the results of those who used other osteoarthritis treatments—both conventional pharmaceuticals and nutritional approaches. To accomplish this properly, the study had to be a suitable length. It also had to include the standard scientific assays and testing measures that are used in double-blind studies of pharmaceutical drugs. According to Dr. Miller, "The criteria we used to determine whether SierraSil worked were identical to the best testing methods employed by pharmaceutical firms." He further explained, "It was a standardized approach at the highest level. Very few companies that sell dietary, nutritional, or herbal supplements submit their products to this type of process and investigation. In fact, most dietary and nutriceutical supplements do not undergo this type of research at all. Usually the manufacturers of such products just rely on anecdotal information."

In developing the study, Dr. Miller and his colleagues began with an in-depth analysis of the published scientific literature on osteoarthritis treatments. They also analyzed the best possible testing standards to use in their study. Based on this analysis, they devised a randomized placebo-controlled double-blind study that was conducted in three research centers. The subjects came from one of the three centers in an effort to achieve evenness of distribution among those who received actual treatments and those in the placebo group. In addition, the fact that the study was double-blind meant that neither the physicians nor the test subjects knew which treatment, if any, they were receiving.

Most of the 107 participants were between fifty and fifty-two years of age; 68 percent were women and 32 percent were men. All of the participants suffered from osteoarthritis of the knee. Great care was taken to ensure that all of the subjects had similar levels of the disease. The study was conducted over a two-month period. "Two months is standard in terms of evaluating a chronic disease like osteoarthritis," according to Dr. Miller, "and the study's population of test subjects ensured that the results achieved were statistically significant."

During the study, the participants were divided into four groups. Each group was given daily doses of one of the following: the SierraSil mineral complex in a high dose, the SierraSil minerals in a low dose, SierraSil in combination with Vincaria, or a placebo. Each participant was assigned to one of the treatment groups according to a randomization chart created by a statistician. The bottles containing the test supplements as well as the placebo were labeled and packaged in such a way that they could not be distinguished from each other. None of the monitoring physicians knew the type of supplement the participants were receiving.

During the first week of the study, all of the participants were evaluated using x-rays, blood tests, and other diagnostic testing methods. Follow-up tests were administered after two, four, six, and eight weeks, at the study's conclusion. Throughout the study, all of the participants were monitored in terms of their overall body function, pain, and joint stiffness.

Dr. Miller noted, "The clinical trial revealed some very interesting trends. The most important was that we found the SierraSil minerals provided significant benefits within two weeks of being administered. Normally, it may take two months or longer before any degree of improvement is achieved using nutritional supplements. This is true even with glucosamine, which is the gold standard in the nutriceutical industry." In fact, such rapid results as those produced by the SierraSil powder are unheard of when compared to other natural supplements, including chondroitin, MSM, and glucosamine, which typically require at least two months for their benefits to be noticed.

What Dr. Miller and his colleagues found among the study participants who were given SierraSil—regardless of the dosage size or whether Vincaria was included—were statistically significant improvements in each of the three main areas of evaluation: pain, joint stiffness, and overall physical activity and body function. In each of these areas, the participants who took the SierraSil minerals began to exhibit improvements within the first week, with significant changes occurring within two weeks. These improvements continued to increase steadily throughout the rest of the two-month study period.

SUMMATION OF THE STUDIES

SierraSil's extensive testing for safety and effectiveness met with impressive, statistically significant results. Based on the study findings, Dr. Miller concluded, "The SierraSil minerals have been through a battery of tests, including safety tests and human clinical trials, and it has come through with flying colors. In light of the research that has been conducted on the SierraSil minerals, I am comfortable in saying that people with osteoarthritis and a wide range of other types of joint dysfunctions can safely supplement with the SierraSil minerals for years." Given the clinical evidence, it is also evident that the SierraSil minerals act as "a very good anti-inflammatory agent," according to Dr. Miller.

What makes Dr. Miller's statements so impressive is that when he was approached by the Bentleys to conduct the studies, he was highly skeptical of their anecdotal reports, including Peter Bentley's personal experience. "I really didn't think the SierraSil minerals would work," he said, "and I was certainly surprised with the results that we found, particularly in the clinical human trials, where the benefits were achieved so rapidly and unequivocally."

As researchers and health practitioners with a particular interest in natural approaches to health and healing, we shared Dr. Miller's initial skepticism when we first learned about the SierraSil minerals. However, after examining the results of the studies conducted by Dr. Miller, we were forced to change our minds. Furthermore, when we began to see the positive results of SierraSil first-hand (discussed in Chapter 4), we were convinced that this "mineral miracle" did, indeed, work.

Yes, we are impressed with the effects of SierraSil. However, if you suffer from inflammatory pain and are presently taking medication, do not simply stop taking it. If you are worried about potential side effects, voice your concerns to your physician or healthcare provider. He or she can give you information on the risks versus the benefits of that particular treatment, and offer guidance on other medications that may have a better safety profile for your particular condition. Discuss the possibility of taking SierraSil, perhaps along with your current treatment. Many of our colleagues have added SierraSil to both prescription and over-the-counter drug recommendations for their patients. This has resulted in a reduction or complete elimination of the pharmaceutical treatments.

Never be afraid to ask questions. Most MDs and healthcare providers will be more than happy to address your questions or concerns, or refer you to information resources that can.

CONCLUSION

Due to their strong belief in SierraSil, coupled by their willingness to underwrite the necessary scientific studies, the Bentleys are now able to offer new hope to anyone who suffers from arthritis and other painful inflammatory health conditions.

Safety and toxicity studies proved that SierraSil is safe for long-term use. The results of the mechanism of action study showed that this mineral complex is able to prevent the breakdown of cartilage. More important, its anti-inflammatory properties can actually stop inflammation—the primary cause of rheumatoid arthritis, osteoarthritis, and a host of other chronic degenerative illnesses.

The human clinical trials showed that SierraSil works, and that it works rapidly in supporting noticeable and significant improvements in joint pain and stiffness. Not only does this unique mineral composition appear to alleviate chronic inflammation more quickly than other natural supplements, it also does so with well-documented safety.

Now that you are aware of the impressive scientific evidence supporting the safety and effectiveness of SierraSil, it is time to examine this natural supplement's full range of health benefits. This is the focus of Chapter 4.

CHAPTER 4

Understanding the Health Benefits of SierraSil

In Chapter 3, you learned that the SierraSil mineral complex not only acts quickly to ease both rheumatoid and osteoarthritis pain—usually within two weeks or less—but also acts to reverse the destructive processes involved in the breakdown and loss of cartilage. You also learned how SierraSil inhibits the various genes that are responsible for creating chronic inflammation in the body—genes that are culprits in a wide-range of degenerative diseases. The SierraSil compound, therefore, may potentially benefit chronic degenerative health problems well beyond arthritis and other joint disorders.

In this chapter, we will explain why we believe that SierraSil will prove to be an important weapon in your nutritional arsenal when it comes to supporting both the prevention of chronic degenerative disease and the alleviation of its symptoms. First, we will share author Dr. Shari Lieberman's personal experiences using SierraSil, as well as the experiences of some of our colleagues. Then, we will explore chronic inflammation, examining both its mechanism and its role in the development of a variety of disorders. Finally, we will discover how SierraSil can relieve the problem of chronic inflammation.

AN AUTHOR'S PERSONAL ACCOUNT

As recognized leaders in the growing field of nutritionally based approaches to healing, we constantly receive news about so-called "breakthrough" supplements. While there certainly are exciting developments in this field, few of the claims made about "miracle" products are backed by studies, and few products live up to their claims. That's why when we consider a new supplement, we first read the studies behind it. Then, even if the studies appear sound, we test the supplement on ourselves or on chronic sufferers whom we can observe. It is only under these conditions that we can fully and impartially evaluate the effectiveness of the supplement.

As it happened, when Dr. Lieberman first learned about the SierraSil mineral compound, she was experiencing back and hip pain, and was seeking relief. Based on the research that was shared with her about SierraSil—research that we present in Chapter 3— she decided to see if supplementation with these minerals would prove helpful. Here is what happened.

Dr. Lieberman's Words

Within the last year, I sustained an injury to my hip. As a result, I developed severe inflammation in the surrounding area and was in a great deal of pain. The pain became so acute that I eventually resorted to using Bextra after several natural health approaches failed to bring me the relief I sought.

I did not want to take Bextra for more than a few weeks—just long enough to get me past the most severe pain. Then shortly after I started taking it, information was released about how dangerous Bextra and related drugs were when taken long-term. Also, the pain relief I experienced from Bextra was only moderate. Obviously, the decision to stop at that point was simple.

It was around this time that I became aware of the SierraSil complex and the research that supported its use. Based on the scientific studies I read, I decided to try SierraSil myself. Because of the severity of my pain, I took five capsules of the powder once a day. To my surprise, it worked remarkably well. Within two weeks, my pain subsided to the point where I could start exercising again. Even my modified exercise did not exacerbate the pain and inflammation I had been experiencing. Instead, SierraSil allowed me to heal without staying off my feet (which is impossible for me anyway!). After a few months, I cut down to a maintenance dose of three capsules per day.

Given what I know about the time it takes for most nutritional supplements to take effect and provide noticeable benefits, I was impressed by the speed with which SierraSil worked for me. As a result, I have continued taking three SierraSil capsules per day. I take them in the middle of the day, away from any other supplements that contain calcium so that they don't interfere with the SierraSil compound's absorption. I can also say that when I travel for a week or so and I forget to take SierraSil—yes, I can forget to take my supplements too!—I start to feel a little ache in my hip or my lower back. That ache goes away as soon as I again start taking the capsules.

HEALERS HEAL THEMSELVES

As you can see, health professionals are definitely not immune to physical pain. So when drugs and natural products don't work, we feel as frustrated as any patient in the same position. However, when we *do* find something that works well, we are in an excellent position to spread the word. What follows are the stories of two colleagues who have used the SierraSil mineral compound to treat joint and muscle pain.

Dr. James LaValle's Experience

James LaValle, RPh, ND, CCN, is a leading expert in naturopathic medicine and a certified clinical nutritionist, as well as a nationally renowned pharmacist who was recognized by *American Druggist* as one of the "50 Most Influential Druggists" for his work promoting natural medicine. Dr. LaValle is also the co-founder of the Living Longer Institute, an integrative medical clinic in Cincinnati, Ohio, and Adjunct Assistant Professor at the University of Cincinnati College of Pharmacy, where he teaches students about nutrition and the use of herbal medicine. He is also a recognized authority in the field of sports medicine. Moreover, Dr. LaValle has had firsthand experience with the benefits of SierraSil.

79

Dr. LaValle's Words

I use the SierraSil mineral compound because I train a lot. In fact, I have close to thirty years experience with strength training and conditioning at an elite level. In addition to training professional athletes, I am a professional athlete myself, and compete in weight lifting competitions and other sports events.

As a result of my rigorous exercise and weight-training regimen, I recently developed some problems with my lower back, in the sense that it was becoming inflamed and beginning to disrupt part of my life. I also started to experience pain in my hip. Knowing that my problem was due to inflammation, I immediately began a nutritional supplementation program specifically geared to reduce inflammation. This included high doses of MSM of up to 10 to 15 grams per day, as well as glucosamine and natural herbal COX-2 inhibitors such as tumeric and curcumin extracts. On particularly bad days, I would even use Celebrex, although I mostly avoided drugs because of their potential side effects.

My nutritional regimen helped take the edge off of my back and hip pain, but still did not provide me with the degree of relief I was looking for. Then I learned about SierraSil and, based on the studies I read, I started to take it. It produced results very quickly, significantly reducing my inflammation and making a big difference in my comfort level. The other products definitely helped, but not to the degree that SierraSil did, and I continue to supplement with it each day.

Based on my background as both a research pharmacist and a naturopathic physician, I believe that SierraSil has proven to be effective for me because it is a very rich trace mineral nutrient. Most people in the United States have a low mineral status, especially with regard to trace minerals. Our bodies run on enzymes, and enzymes need trace minerals in order to function appropriately. Without an adequate supply of trace minerals, the enzymes responsible for regulating inflammation and tissue repair are unable to do their job. This leads to disruptions in the body's repair processes, as well in the cycling of collagen. The trace mineral blend in SierraSil helps to fuel those enzymes to regulate the inflammatory process, and also to regulate the breakdown of collagen so that the body's joints, ligaments, and tendons are able to restore themselves. There are other natural products that do this to some degree, but they don't work as quickly as SierraSil does.

The fact that the SierraSil formulation contains extracts of cat's claw is also interesting. Cat's claw helps to regulate the inflammatory process that underlies so many chronic health problems, so adding cat's claw to SierraSil creates a synergistic effect by combining the trace minerals with a proven botanical that also regulates inflammation. It's an elegant formula that acts like a one-two punch to address one of the most common health complaints today.

Dr. Clement Williams' Experience

A physician and surgeon, Clement Williams, MD, has been practicing medicine for more than forty years. Currently, he serves as the director of the Dundarave Medical Clinic in West Vancouver, British Columbia, and specializes in using anti-aging medicine in combination with proper nutrition and exercise. Below, you'll learn what he has to say about the SierraSil mineral compound.

Dr. Williams' Words

I have a fused right knee and a left knee in which cartilage was removed about two years ago. At the time, X-rays revealed evidence of early osteoarthritis. Sometime later, I compounded this problem with a knee injury. It became so painful that walking from my desk to examine my patients was difficult, and this was only a distance of three steps. To relieve the pain, I tried a number of prescription pain relievers, but they didn't work. Instead, my pain continued to get worse.

Around that time, I learned about SierraSil. When told of its potential benefits, initially I was skeptical, yet the fact that it is a natural product was attractive to me, so I decided to try it. To my surprise, within a week, I began to notice definite benefits. As of this writing, I have been using SierraSil for about one year and am now able to walk pain-free. In fact, I don't experience any pain at all unless I badly overwork my knees. I am very impressed with the results I have achieved, and will continue to take the SierraSil mineral complex.

Since my success using SierraSil, I have begun to recommend it to my patients. They, too, have experienced positive results, usually very quickly. Most report noticeable benefits in less than ten days, while other natural joint support formulas can take up to three months to work. The other thing that greatly impresses me about SierraSil is that it causes absolutely no side effects. It is completely safe, is highly beneficial, and in my opinion should be used by anyone who suffers from arthritis or joint pain.

Now that you have read about Dr. Lieberman's experience with the SierraSil mineral compound, as well as the experience of Drs. LaValle and Williams, let's discuss chronic inflammation and the significant role that it plays not only in rheumatoid and osteoarthritis, but also in a wide range of other serious degenerative disease conditions.

UNDERSTANDING THE PROBLEM OF CHRONIC INFLAMMATION

As explained in Chapter 3, one of the primary mechanisms of action of the SierraSil mineral complex is its suppression of those genes responsible for triggering and perpetuating chronic inflammation. This is why we find SierraSil to be such an exceptional natural alternative to pain relievers and other medications meant to treat arthritis and other inflammation-related disorders. In our view, SierraSil is a superior treatment choice for arthritis and joint pain, not only because it is much safer than pain relievers and other arthritis drugs, but also because it targets and reverses the primary mechanism behind all types of arthritis—inflammation. This is something most arthritis drugs are unable to do. At best, all that such medications can do is provide relief from arthritis pain *symptoms*, not its *cause*.

Because of the way in which SierraSil acts to support the inhibition of chronic inflammation, we believe that its potential benefits as a health supplement go far beyond the alleviation of arthritis and joint pain. Why? Because, as a growing body of scientific research makes abundantly clear, chronic inflammation is a primary cause of or contributing factor to most of the chronic degenerative diseases that are responsible for our nation's current health crisis. To understand this, we first must understand the inflammatory process itself.

What Is Inflammation?

Inflammation was designed by nature to act as an important yet temporary healing response whenever the body is injured through trauma; is exposed to infectious microorganisms, such as bacteria, fungi, and viruses; or is exposed to allergy-causing triggers (allergens). During such situations, inflammation is absolutely essential for the proper repair of injured bones, joints, organs, or tissues, and for the restoration of health following infection or exposure to allergens.

To understand a healthy inflammatory response, consider what happens when you cut yourself. As soon as the cut occurs, your immune system rushes into action, directing various proteins and other healing agents to the site of the cut in order to seal it off from potential infection. Should foreign bodies be present, immune cells known as macrophages are also directed to the cut, where they go to work literally devouring the microorganisms before they can cause any harm. Other immune agents are also activated in order to eliminate waste byproducts and other cellular debris caused by the immune response. As a result of these activities, the area of the cut usually reddens and swells as you experience sensations of heat and pain. Once the cut begins to heal, however, a healthy immune system recognizes that its task has been accomplished, and the inflammatory response stops. Soon thereafter, the swelling, heat, and pain begin to subside as the cut continues to mend and, finally, heals altogether.

Immune activities such as the one described above are known as *acute inflammation* responses and represent vital defense reactions on the part of your body. In addition to heat, redness, pain, and swelling, episodes of acute inflammation can also result in a temporary loss of function in the affected part of your body. Acute inflammation is usually very short-lived, however, lasting no more than a few days in most cases. But when inflammation lasts longer, becoming chronic, the stage is set for potential health problems to arise, some of which can be quite serious, and even life-threatening.

What is *chronic inflammation*? It is a low-grade ongoing or recurrent condition that occurs when the immune system perceives itself to being under continuous attack. In some cases, this perception is accurate, due to a variety of external causes discussed below. But in many other cases, chronic inflammation is due to what is called an *autoimmune response* in which the immune system attacks other parts of the body—joints, organs, and/or tissues—inappropriately. Instead of resulting in healing, as happens in the case of acute inflammation, chronic inflammation produces symptoms of pain and swelling that either occur continuously, or repeatedly and intermittently flare up.

In some cases of chronic inflammation, there are no obvious symptoms of the problem, and the individual continues to feel fine. But inside the body, internal scarring may occur, setting the stage for eventual degenerative disease. In fact, people can remain unaware that they have a developing health problem for years before serious symptoms present themselves. In the case of heart attack—which strikes approximately 50 percent of sufferers without warning—the first obvious symptoms, such as chest pain and shortness of breath, are usually preceded by years of slow-burning inflammation of the artery linings.

According to Nancy Appleton, PhD, author of *Stopping Inflammation: Relieving the Cause of Degenerative Diseases*, although chronic inflammation can be caused by the body's failure to shut down the process of acute inflammation once it has done its job, many cases of chronic inflammation develop on their own. That is, these cases develop without any initial acute symptoms, and therefore are not detected until a far more serious condition makes itself known.

Causes of Chronic Inflammation

Chronic inflammation can be caused by a variety of factors. The one common denominator among all causes of chronic inflammation is that the immune system perceives itself to be under attack. According to Dr. Appleton, causes of chronic inflammation include the following:

❏ *Allergies and sensitivities.* Allergic reactions to foods, food sensitivities, and allergies to environmental substances such as chemicals and dander can cause the immune system to initiate an inflammatory response that can damage the body's tissues.

❏ *Advanced glycation end products (AGEs).* AGEs are a class of complex, often unstable reactive compounds formed in the body under certain conditions, such as when certain foods are eaten or when excess sugar occurs in the bloodstream. These compounds can initiate a wide range of abnormal responses in cells and tissues, causing or contributing to a variety of disorders, including not only inflammation itself, but also Alzheimer's disease, arthritis, atherosclerosis, cataracts, diabetes, high blood pressure, kidney disease, and macular degeneration.

❏ *Environmental toxins.* Today, the average person in the United States is said to carry at least 700 different types of toxic chemicals in his or her cells and tissues, due to the increasing glut of toxic chemicals that are introduced to our air, soil, and water supplies each and every year. When such chemical toxins gain a foothold in the body, inflammation can occur in the body's attempt to dislodge and eliminate them.

❏ *Estrogen therapy.* The use of conventional estrogen therapy has been shown to cause both chronic inflammation and unhealthy blood clotting.

❏ *Fatigue.* When fatigue becomes chronic, it places stress on the body. This, in turn, can lead to chronic inflammation as the body tries to cope with a prolonged lack of energy.

❏ *Free radical damage.* Free radicals are atoms or groups of atoms that have at least one unpaired electron, and are therefore unstable. When free radicals occur within the body, they ricochet wildly, damaging cells and contributing to inflammation and the progression of cancer, heart disease, and other disorders.

❏ *Hypertension.* Hypertension, or high blood pressure, is known to amplify the inflammatory response.

❏ *Infectious microorganisms.* Infectious bacteria, fungi, parasites, and viruses trigger the immune system to secrete various immune cells. If left unchecked, these cells can cause damage to healthy body tissue, leading to chronic inflammation.

❏ *Obesity.* Because fat cells release cytokines—chemical substances that produce inflammation—obesity has a causal relationship to inflammation. As you might predict, the more obese a person is, the higher his or her degree of inflammation is likely to be.

❏ *Physical injury.* Injuries such as burns, bruises, fractures, and sprains—as well as damage caused by excessive cold, ionizing radiation, and ultraviolet light exposure—can cause or exacerbate chronic inflammation.

❏ *Smoking.* Due to the chemicals present in tobacco, smoking—as well as regular exposure to secondhand smoke—is another common cause of inflammation.

❏ *Surgery.* Acute inflammation is a normal response to surgical procedures. But in many cases, the inflammatory response becomes chronic due to one of the other factors in this list.

❏ *Vaccinations.* Vaccines, which are used to protect against various illnesses, cause the production of interferon gamma, a protein that can lead to chronic inflammation.

Now you know some of the causes of chronic inflammation. But before we can discuss the role it plays in certain chronic degenerative diseases, it's necessary to take another look at the inflammatory process, this time focusing in on what occurs when inflammation becomes chronic.

When the Inflammatory Response Becomes Chronic

The inflammatory response is initiated by the release of tissue hormones called histamines and blood proteins called kinins, which cause blood vessel dilation, increased blood flow, and tissue swelling. Very quickly, the release of other chemicals also occurs, creating an internal flood of cytokines, eosinophils, prostaglandins, leukotrienes, and interleukin, all of which advance the progression of the inflammatory response, causing the tissues to further swell and heat up.

As this process continues to unfold, cells known as *circulating immune complexes,* or *CICs,* are produced. CICs are composed of *antigens*—bacteria, toxins, and other cells that pose a threat to the body; and *antibodies*—protein substances produced by the body in response to specific antigens. In cases of acute inflammation, the body is able to easily eliminate CICs from the body via the liver. In cases of chronic inflammation, though, the buildup of CICs can become too great, eventually overwhelming both the liver and the immune system. When this happens, liver and immune functions become compromised. If this process continues unchecked, other organs can be affected as well, setting the stage for a variety of degenerative diseases to develop as the CICs become lodged in the body. According to Dr. Appleton:

> An individual's genetic blueprint will determine where CICs may lodge. If there is a weakness somewhere in the body, the immune system will attack that location. Inflammation will move right into the unhealthy area to attempt healing. Macrophages (a class of white blood cells that hunt invaders) may act as a secondary line of defense, attacking CICs in the bloodstream or in the lungs. If CICs are not removed, they may trigger a cascade of events that lead to multiple symptoms, and sometimes tissue damage.

People who suffer from nutritional deficiencies have a greater risk of developing CICs that defy the body's attempts to eliminate them. This is particularly true when someone is deficient in trace minerals, which are essential for catalyzing so many of the body's self-regulatory mechanisms. And when CICs remain in the body, the person becomes especially susceptible to developing one or more of the degenerative health conditions that—although they may seem unrelated to one another—are all largely due to chronic low-grade inflammation.

INFLAMMATION AND HEART DISEASE

Now that you know a little more about chronic inflammation, it's time to learn how this problem plays a major role in the development of heart disease, including heart attack.

The link between inflammation and heart disease was first established in the late nineteenth century by German physiologist Rudolph Virchow, whose research indicated that the primary cause of heart disease was inflammation of the arteries and the heart muscle itself. Dr. Virchow's research was confirmed by his examination of the hearts of people who had died of heart disease. He found that the hearts looked as if they had been bruised, battered, and infected.

Unfortunately, Dr. Virchow's findings were ignored throughout most of the twentieth century, as cardiologists focused instead on cholesterol levels and cholesterol-lowering drugs, such as the popular class of drugs known as statins. (See the inset on page 91 to learn more about statins.) It was not until the 1980s that researchers again considered the role that inflammation plays in heart disease. One of those researchers was Dr. Peter Libby, a professor of medicine at Harvard University's Medical School. Dr. Libby confirmed the role that inflammation plays in causing heart disease by introducing bacterial toxins into the arterial cells of rats. The rats' bodies then released cytokines as part of the inflammatory process. When Dr. Libby examined human tissues taken from people who suffered from heart disease, he found levels of cytokines similar to those elevated levels found in the rats. His scientific paper *Cytokines in the Pathogenesis of Atherosclerosis*, published in 2002, is one of a number of research papers that clearly confirm the principal role inflammation plays in the onset and progression of heart disease.

Another study, known as the Harvard University's Health Study, published in 1999, compared 534 men who had suffered heart attacks with an equal number of men who had not. All of the men in the heart attack group had levels of inflammation much higher than levels in the non-heart attack group, leading researchers to conclude that chronic inflammation increases the risk of heart attack by at least 300 percent, and increases the risk of stroke by at least 200 percent. These and similar studies linking inflammation to heart disease have substantiated Dr. Virchow's observations of more than a century ago.

How Inflammation Can Lead to Heart Disease

Conventional wisdom holds that most heart disease is caused by elevated levels of cholesterol building up inside the *lumen*—the inner cavity—of our arteries. This elevated traveling cholesterol accumulation, which comes from both diet and genetically driven liver synthesis, is called *stable plaque*. Stable plaques begins forming in the body around the age of ten, and gradually adhere to any portions of the arteries that have been injured due to exposure to environmental pollutants, high blood pressure, smoking, stress, diabetes, poor diet, or obesity. Looking like a "fatty streak," the plaque clogs the lumen, and depending on the extent of the blockage, may cause angina (heart pain) or a complete loss of oxygen to the heart muscle (heart attack). Coronary bypass surgery or angioplasty can help relieve the symptoms of stable plaque formation. The problem is that this traditional model for heart disease is only 30 percent of the story. The remaining causes of heart disease—70 percent of the story—are primarily associated with chronic inflammation.

Inflammation plays a significant role in nearly 1.9 million cardiac-related deaths each year in the United States. How does inflammation accomplish its deadly mission? It does so in part by associating itself with a type of cholesterol called low density lipoprotein (LDL-C). LDL-C becomes dangerous when it penetrates the lining of the artery walls and is deposited in the wall itself—not in the lumen, where stable plaque is found. Since LDL does not belong in the artery wall, the body perceives it as an invader or a foreign body. As you would expect, the immune system sends cells called macrophages to clear the LDL from the artery. The macrophages then engulf the trapped LDL and in the process release inflammatory substances. This engagement causes the laying down of a frothy looking complex inside the artery walls. Because of its appearance, this LDL, macrophage, inflammatory complex is often referred to as a *foam cell*. And when many foam cells accumulate inside the artery, they form a lipid-laden core called *vulnerable plaque*. It is this vulnerable plaque that is two and a half times more deadly and sinister then the traditional stable plaque. Why? Due to triggers ranging from body movement to simple heartbeat rhythm, stress, or infection, vulnerable plaque can rupture without warning, causing its contents—including substances that cause blood clotting—to spill out into the bloodstream. The resulting blockage can, in turn, lead to angina, heart attack, and stroke.

Compounding this problem is the fact that, unlike stable plaques, vulnerable plaques are often not detected by traditional cardiovascular diagnostic tests because they do not push into the artery lumen until they are nearly 40 percent the size of the artery's circumference. In other words, when a vulnerable plaque is big enough for detection, it's often too late for you. That is why many people who are not diagnosed with blocked arteries nevertheless suffer heart attacks.

In addition to heart attack and stroke, chronic inflammation and the resultant vulnerable plaque it forms can also cause or exacerbate other forms of heart disease, including angina, congestive heart failure, coronary stenosis, and high blood pressure. The important lesson here is that the old model of heart disease, which focused primarily on cholesterol levels and stable plaque development, is only a third of the story. Today, we know the importance of aggressively preventing and reversing the buildup of chronic inflammation and vulnerable plaque. Doing so can literally save your life.

INFLAMMATION AND CANCER

An increasing number of physicians and researchers now recognize that, in addition to playing a major role in heart disease, inflammation also plays a role in the development and progression of cancer.

Once again, we find that Dr. Rudolph Virchow, a nineteenth-century physiologist, was one of the first to suggest a link between

Statin Drugs—The Good, the Bad, and the Ugly

Currently, statin drugs, as a class, are the medications most commonly prescribed by physicians to lower cholesterol and protect against heart disease. Emerging scientific research clearly suggests that statins also provide anti-inflammatory benefits, and that it is this activity, more than their cholesterol-lowering effects, that can make them so effective for treating and protecting against heart disease. There is little doubt that statins can significantly reduce the incidence of heart disease and death caused by heart attack and stroke, especially for people who have a high risk of developing cardiovascular illness. This is particularly true for people who have already experienced a heart attack, as well as for those who have undergone angioplasty or bypass surgery, even if their overall cholesterol levels are low.

In one study, which examined over 1,600 patients who had been hospitalized for heart disease, including heart attack, it was found that when statin use was discontinued, patients were nearly three times as likely to suffer from a recurrence of their heart problems as were patients who continued to use statin drugs. Such research clearly points out the potential benefits statin drugs can provide for people with heart disease.

In addition to lowering cholesterol and helping to protect the body against chronic inflammation, other benefits of statin drugs have been known to include:

❏ Stabilizing vulnerable plaque

❏ Improving blood function in a way similar to nitric oxide

❏ Reducing and reversing arterial calcification

❏ Reducing the risk of stroke

❏ Reducing the risk of bone fracture and osteoporosis

❏ Improving macular degeneration

❏ Protecting against sepsis and septic shock

Preliminary research suggests that statins may also prove to have benefits for certain types of cancer, such as colon and prostate cancer, as well as for HIV and even Alzheimer's disease.

Not all of the news about statins is good, however. Like all other drugs, statins can cause side effects. Some of these side effects are not necessarily serious—generalized feelings of soreness, for example. But in severe cases, the muscle cells of people who use statins can break down and release myoglobin, an iron-containing protein, into the blood, potentially leading to impaired kidney function and even kidney failure. In addition, statins can inhibit the body's ability to produce coenzyme Q_{10} (CoQ_{10}), an essential nutrient that is vital for healthy heart function, and can even deplete CoQ_{10} from the muscles—including the heart muscle—eventually resulting in death.

Statins can also compromise liver function and cause problems such as peripheral neuropathy, an inflammatory condition that involves damage to the peripheral nervous system. In people with low levels of LDL cholesterol, statins can also interfere with the brain's neurotransmitters, leading to episodes of amnesia that can last anywhere from a few minutes to several hours. Ironically, it was reported in the medical journal *Circulation* that statins can even cause congestive heart failure, an extremely serious condition. In fact, a growing number of cardiologists now believe that the overuse of statins is one of the major reasons that there has been an increased incidence of congestive heart failure in the United States over the past decade.

Finally, be aware that many of the benefits of statins listed earlier—the stabilizing of vulnerable plaque, for instance—occur at higher doses of the drugs. And it is these higher doses that are associated with abnormal liver function and muscle cell breakdown.

Based on the pros and cons of statin use, some experts advise that statins be prescribed only for people who have a history of serious heart disease, including an incidence of heart attack or heart surgeries such as angioplasty, bypass, or the insertion of a stent. In such cases, these experts further advise that patients supplement with at least 50 to 100 milligrams of soluble CoQ_{10} to prevent this vital nutrient from being depleted by prolonged stain use.

A more conservative approach is recommended for people who have no history of heart disease. For them, experts often advise a healthy diet and exercise program, as well as supplementation with natural anti-inflammatory nutrients, including fish oil and the SierraSil mineral compound. (To learn more about supplementation, see Chapter 5.)

cancer and inflammation. In Virchow's view, cancer was due to irritation at the cellular level that triggered inflammation and the excessive growth associated with cancer. But just as Virchow's views regarding inflammation and heart disease were ignored with the dawn of cholesterol-lowering drugs, his views on the cause of cancer were ignored once researchers started to explore the use of chemotherapy and radiation to treat cancer, and to study the relationship between genes and cancer. In recent years, however, Virchow's cancer theory has been vindicated. In 2001, for example, Dr. Angus Dalgleish and other researchers at the University of Leicester's Department of Oncology in England, presented findings indicating that the most important cause of cancer is prolonged overactivation of the immune system, which, as we have discussed, results in chronic inflammation. In their paper, published in the *British Journal of Cancer,* Dalgleish and his colleagues termed tissues in the body affected by inflammation "a melting pot of cancer-causing molecules." Dalgleish stated that according to his research, there are elevated levels of C-reactive protein (CRP)—an indicator of inflammation—in most types of cancer, including cancer of the breast, colon, lung, pancreas, and prostate.

Other investigators have since confirmed the findings of Dr. Dalgleish and his colleagues, identifying chronic inflammation as an important trigger for the development of solid cancer tumors. One of these researchers is Dr. Lisa Coussens of the Cancer Research Institute at the University of California at San Francisco. "Tumors, when they're developing, are just proliferating cells," Dr Coussens explains. "The theory is that this is much like a wound to the host [the body]. So inflammatory cells come in and do their job. They urge the growth [cancer] onward." Additional studies have also found a strong associative link between inflammation and chromosome damage and cellular proliferation, both of which are hallmarks of cancer. In addition, once cancer starts to take hold in the body, it has been found that chronic inflammation can interfere with the natural defenses that might otherwise keep the cancer in check.

Researchers are still investigating the link between chronic inflammation and cancer, and have yet to explain the precise mechanism by which a prolonged inflammatory response can cause and further the spread of cancer. Based on current findings, however, there is no doubt that inflammation *does* play a significant role in cancer growth. Therefore, reversing chronic inflammation appears to be an essential step in both the prevention and the cure of cancer.

INFLAMMATION AND OTHER DISEASE CONDITIONS

Heart disease and cancer are only two of the many conditions that, according to research, are caused or exacerbated by chronic inflammation. What follows is a list of other disorders that either have been causally linked to inflammation—meaning that inflammation is believed to be at the heart of the problem—or have inflammation as a component.

❏ Alzheimer's disease

❏ Blood sugar problems, including hyper- and hypoglycemia

❏ Candidiasis

❏ Cystic fibrosis

❏ Epilepsy

❏ Headache, including migraines

❏ Heartburn

❏ Inflammatory bowel disease, including irritable bowel syndrome (IBS), Crohn's disease, and ulcerative colitis

❏ Kidney disease

❏ Parkinson's disease

❏ Respiratory conditions

As time goes on, researchers may link chronic inflammation with additional health disorders. But even now, we know enough about the effects of inflammation to realize the importance of identifying inflammation in the body, and finding a way to treat it. The remainder of this chapter addresses both of these issues.

IDENTIFYING INFLAMMATION

At this point, you are probably asking yourself how can you determine whether or not you suffer from chronic, low-grade inflammation, especially since common diagnostic tests—cholesterol tests, EKGs, and the like—do not screen for inflammation. Fortunately, there exists a simple and inexpensive test that can quickly determine the level of inflammation in your body. It is known as a CRP blood test and is readily available throughout the country.

Earlier in this chapter, mention was made of CRP, which stands for *C-reactive protein,* a type of protein that is present in trace amounts in the blood of healthy people, and in higher amounts in people suffering from chronic inflammation. CRP is produced by the liver in response to invading pathogens and toxins, as well as during chronic states of inflammation. As a result, CRP is considered an accurate marker of inflammation.

Determining your CRP levels can be a vital part of protecting yourself against a wide variety of chronic disease conditions. This is particularly true of heart disease. Physicians now regard elevated CRP levels to be a better indicator of high heart disease risk than elevated levels of total cholesterol, LDL cholesterol, and the amino acid homocysteine. In fact, higher-than-normal CRP levels can increase your risk of heart disease—especially heart attack, angina, and stroke—by as much as 400 to 800 percent.

Because inflammation can lead to disorders other than heart disease, it's not surprising to learn that high CRP levels are also associated with a higher risk of Alzheimer's disease, arthritis, cancer, diabetes (Type II), hyperglycemia, hypertension, lupus, obesity, periodontal disease, and Syndrome X, a cluster of disorders that have been linked to insulin resistance. High levels of CRP are even considered a predictor of complications following organ transplant surgery.

THE EFFECTS OF SIERRASIL ON INFLAMMATION

Although extensive scientific studies evaluating the effects of the SierraSil mineral compound on levels of C-reactive protein have yet to be conducted, initial observations indicate that regular supplementation with SierraSil can help maintain lower-than-normal levels of CRP.

Based on the positive reports he received from patients who used SierraSil, Dr. Clement Williams—director of Dundarave Medical Clinic in West Vancouver, British Columbia—decided to conduct CRP blood tests on nine patients, all of whom had been taking 1 to 3 grams (1,000–3,000 milligrams) of SierraSil for two years or longer. The results of the tests were impressive.

The normal range for CRP in healthy people is less than 5.0 milligrams per liter of blood (5.0 mg/L). "If the test shows a value greater than 5 mg per liter," Dr. Williams says, "this is a red light which tells us that there is some serious disease hiding somewhere in the body, of which both the patient and the doctor were unaware." Of the patients he tested, Dr. Williams reports that their CRP levels ranged from 0.9 to 4.8 milligrams per liter, with the average being 2.2 milligrams per liter.

Commenting on these remarkable findings, Dr. Williams says, "I am really impressed with the results. All of the patients' CRP levels are in the low normal range, a strong indication that they are in overall good health. In addition to their low CRP levels, all of these patients have enjoyed the benefits that SierraSil provides for relief of arthritis pain, with absolutely no side effects. All and all, I find the results my patients are having using SierraSil to be very favorable."

CONCLUSION

After reading this chapter, you should realize the serious threat that chronic inflammation can pose to your health. Compounding the problem is the fact that in many cases, symptoms of chronic inflammation are virtually nonexistent until they flare up in the form of a serious health problem such as heart disease. For this reason, we believe that all of our clients and patients should be screened for chronic inflammation using a C-reactive protein blood test, and that, when necessary, they take steps to get their inflammation under control.

SierraSil and the Gastrointestinal Tract

Many people who use SierraSil to relieve the pain of arthritis report that they have gained relief not only from their arthritis symptoms, but also from digestive problems such as irritable bowel syndrome (IBS) and Crohn's disease. We believe the reason for such improvement is the smectite clay component of SierraSil, along with the additional benefits provided by the various minerals contained in the compound.

As we discussed in Chapter 1, the healing clay contained in the SierraSil mineral complex is believed to promote healthy functioning of the gastrointestinal tract in a variety of ways. Research has shown that clay helps neutralize and eliminate toxins, and that it absorbs viruses and various types of microscopic parasites that can cause disturbances in the gut. It most likely also absorbs the gas caused by improper digestion. Thus, SierraSil may help prevent and alleviate gastrointestinal disorders ranging from bad breath to constipation, diarrhea, diverticulitis, flatulence, food poisoning, irritable bowel syndrome, and more.

Because SierraSil promotes the health of the gut, it may also benefit the entire body by preventing a disorder known as leaky gut syndrome. Leaky gut syndrome occurs when the intestinal lining becomes overly permeable, usually as a result of irritation and inflammation. This condition of heightened permeability allows undigested food particles, as well as bacteria, fungi, viruses, and yeast, to move into the bloodstream, causing havoc. It also allows pathogens outside the gut to enter it, causing gastrointestinal disturbances and disorders such as irritable bowel syndrome. In both of these cases, the immune system springs into action, releasing antibodies, cytokines, histamines, and other substances that, as you know, can trigger your body's inflammatory response. In fact, leaky gut syndrome has been associated with a number of inflammation-related disorders, from allergies to Crohn's disease to rheumatoid arthritis.

Because of the protective and healing properties of smectite clay, as well as the anti-inflammatory activities of the SierraSil mineral compound, we believe that SierraSil may help prevent leaky gut syndrome and the problems associated with it. At this point, anecdotal evidence and preliminary studies on the healing effects of SierraSil and its components are encouraging. Future studies are sure to tell us more about this "mineral miracle."

Fortunately, it is not difficult to control inflammation. The first step, of course, is to begin supplementation with the SierraSil mineral compound. But as effective as SierraSil is for protecting and relieving both chronic inflammation and joint pain, it's important to understand that this powder is not a "magic bullet" solution for creating and maintaining good health. That's why we also advise our clients and patients to follow a practical and powerful dietary, nutritional, and lifestyle program. The next chapter discusses the components of that program, giving you the remaining tools you need to enjoy a healthy pain-free life.

CHAPTER 5

Staying Healthy— A Complete Plan of Action

While the nutrients from the SierraSil mineral deposit offer many anti-pain and anti-inflammatory benefits, they constitute only one of the many answers to the overall ravages of aging and disease, and should not be considered a "magic bullet." In fact, we believe that when it comes to your health, no "magic bullet"—whether natural or pharmaceutical—exists. That's why in this chapter, we share with you a complete self-care plan that will help you first achieve good health and then maintain it for a lifetime.

HOW HEALTHY ARE YOU?

A common misconception held by many people—patients and physicians alike—is that good health is simply the absence of obvious health complaints and disease symptoms. In our experience as healthcare professionals, we often meet individuals who believe and assert that they are as healthy as they can be. Upon closer examination, however, all too often this isn't the case. Although they may not be suffering from any obvious signs of illness, when questioned, they often admit to lacking energy, feeling stiffness in their back and joints, suffering from sluggish digestion, experiencing constant stress, having difficulty getting a good night's sleep, or simply having no zest and enthusiasm for life. While none of these complaints is necessarily due to disease, all of them are signs of *dis-ease,* meaning a lack of harmony and balance.

The "How Healthy Are You?" Quiz

To the right of each point, fill in the most appropriate number from 1 to 5, with 1 indicating that you experience the described feeling or condition rarely; 3, that you experience it occasionally; 5, that you experience it often. Note that there are no right or wrong answers to these questions and no one is going to judge you, so you'll want to answer truthfully to get an honest assessment of your health.

1. You go through each day with abundant energy and enthusiasm for what you are doing. _____

2. You fall asleep easily and sleep deeply. _____

3. You awaken each morning feeling greatly refreshed. _____

4. Each morning, you look forward to the day ahead of you. _____

5. You are within 20 pounds of your ideal body weight. _____

6. You are able to move and stretch your body with ease and flexibility. _____

7. You are physically strong and have good muscle tone. _____

8. You exercise on a regular basis. _____

9. You have a positive, optimistic attitude about your life, and find it enjoyable and rewarding to cope with daily challenges. _____

10. You regularly experience feelings of joy and satisfaction. _____

11. You live and work in healthy environments that support your well-being. _____

12. You have strong and emotionally fulfilling relationships with your family and friends. _____

13. You feel connected to the world around you. _____

Total Points: _____

First add up all the points you assigned to the various questions. If your point total falls below 30, your level of health may be easily compromised, and you should immediately start improving your situation by following the guidelines presented in this chapter. If your point total is between 30 and 50 points, you are healthier than most people, but there is room for improvement because you remain subject to fluctuations in your energy levels and overall health. If your point total is above 50 points, congratulations! You have managed to create a stable health environment for yourself. The guidelines provided in this chapter should help you maintain your health long into the future.

If these symptoms sound familiar to you, you should know that such complaints are common to tens of millions of people in our nation. You should also know that if nothing is done to correct some of these problems, eventually, they may lead to chronic illness.

Why is it that so many people who suffer from the problems mentioned earlier consider themselves healthy? The fact is that we as a nation have forgotten what being healthy means. True health is far more than the absence of disease symptoms. It is a state of abundant energy and physical and emotional well-being, including the regular experience of joy and satisfaction. Based on this definition, where do you rank on the scale of optimal health? To help you answer this question, the inset on pages 100 to 101 presents a simple test that will enable you to discover how healthy you really are. As you answer the questions, note how many attributes of health you are now experiencing or, conversely, how few of them you are enjoying. This test is by no means conclusive, but it does provide you with an easy way to assess your health in general terms, and can also help you determine the areas of your health on which you may need to work.

THE ESSENTIALS FOR OPTIMAL HEALTH

Earlier in this chapter, we discussed how most Americans have forgotten what good health is, and we defined it as physical and emotional well-being. Yet another definition of good health has been provided by the American Holistic Medical Association (AHMA), an organization of holistic physicians founded in 1978 by such visionary doctors as C. Norman Shealy, MD, PhD. According to the AHMA, true health is present only when there is harmony and balance in the "whole person," meaning that he or she has physical health, mental health, and spiritual health.

What do we mean when we refer to each of these levels of health? Physical health refers not only to a healthy body, but also to healthy home and work environments. Mental health involves the regular experience of joy, contentment, and peace of mind, as well as freedom from emotional distress such as chronic anxiety, sorrow, anger, or fear. And spiritual health involves having a sense of connectedness with the Divine—with God, with nature, or with whatever force you identify as the ultimate power.

Your Body's Built-In Mechanism for Maintaining a Healthy Balance

The importance of balance as it relates to good health is wonderfully exemplified by the human body itself in a principle called *homeostasis.* Simply put, homeostasis is the body's inherent capacity to maintain and repair itself by adjusting its various interlinking systems, such as the nervous system, circulatory system, digestive system, immune system, etc. When you are healthy, balance begins to be restored at the first sign of any event that disrupts the body's ability to properly function. For example, should you cut yourself, your body's healing process starts immediately. Signals from the brain set in motion a cascade of events that cause the circulatory system to deliver more oxygen and vital nutrients to the site of the cut, while the immune system creates a temporary state of healthy inflammation to both speed healing and ward off potential pathogens that might otherwise infect the wound. This entire process happens automatically, without the need for an outside influence to set it into motion.

But should you be taxed with, for example, chronic stress, lack of sleep, and/or poor nutrition, your body's ability to repair itself can be impaired, causing the cut to heal more slowly. Because of your body's marvelous design, though, it takes a good many stressors to compromise the process of homeostasis, and even then, the body continues its attempt to heal itself.

Above, we mentioned that inflammation is one of the signs that the body is trying to heal itself. Other possible signs of the body's struggle to restore balance include fever, vomiting, and diarrhea, all of which generally run their course over a short period of time without the need for outside intervention. Unfortunately, the value of such symptoms is often overlooked by conventional physicians, who immediately seek to suppress these signs of the body's efforts to balance itself. As a result, these symptoms are often replaced by problems that pose even greater threats to the body's well-being.

Skilled health practitioners recognize symptoms of the body's self-regulatory system for what they are, and rather than interfering, help the body achieve its goal of regained balance. Only when symptoms become very painful or life-threatening do these doctors consider interrupting the homeostatic process.

From a holistic standpoint, helping the body repair and restore itself means ensuring that a patient's needs are properly addressed for each of the areas mentioned earlier—the body, mind, and spirit. By doing so, physicians not only enhance patients' ability to heal, but also provide them with a new understanding about themselves and their life challenges. For example, if proper diet, appropriate supplementation, and adequate rest help patients relieve hypertension, they may come to recognize how chronic stress at work or at home, along with poor eating habits, contributed to their high blood pressure, and take the steps necessary to avoid repeating their mistakes.

Now that you have a better understanding of homeostasis and you know the three areas of life that can improve or impair your health, let's examine the self-care steps you can take to enjoy the best health possible in these three areas. Please realize that if you or a loved one currently suffers from a serious health problem, you should seek appropriate medical attention immediately. The following principles are not intended to take the place of professional care. However, through both personal experience and the experience of our many clients and patients, we have learned that the following steps can help you make significant and lasting improvements in your overall health and well-being.

As discussed earlier in the chapter, true health is present only when the individual is in balance, and balance is achieved only when he or she is healthy in body, mind, and spirit. In the remainder of this chapter, we'll look at each of these three areas in turn and discuss how you can take steps to create harmonious good health.

CREATING PHYSICAL HEALTH

Our first area of discussion is physical health. As first mentioned on page 102, physical health includes both a healthy body and healthy home and work environments.

Creating a Healthy Body

Five simple yet essential steps are necessary for achieving and maintaining a healthy body. They include:

1. Following a proper diet.

2. Taking adequate nutritional supplementation.

3. Drinking an adequate amount of water.

4. Getting regular exercise.

5. Getting adequate sleep and relaxation.

The scientific evidence that each of these factors plays a critical role in safeguarding our health is truly overwhelming. Unfortunately, as a nation, we are deficient in all of these areas even though each of them, from eating a healthy diet to getting adequate sleep, is well within our grasp. What follows are the basic guidelines you can follow to quickly and easily make these components part of your daily life.

Diet

A healthy diet is the cornerstone of optimal health. Maimonides, the twelfth-century physician, wrote, "No illness which can be treated by diet should be treated by any other means." This sentiment echoed that of Hippocrates, the Father of Western Medicine, who more than a thousand years earlier had said, "Let food be thy medicine, and medicine thy food."

Sadly, today little emphasis is placed on diet and nutrition in our nation's medical schools and universities, with medical students receiving, on average, only four to eight hours of instruction in these areas during their education. As a result, unless they have made an effort to study diet and nutrition on their own, the majority of conventional physicians are unable to guide patients in creating healthy diets. In recent years, there has been a growing awareness of the importance of diet, with groups like the American Medical Association and the American Cancer Society urging us to eat at least five to seven servings of fruits and vegetables each day. Yet recognizing the importance of diet and nutrition is not enough. We also must recognize that each person is unique, with unique nutritional needs based on a number of factors, including age, gender, current health status, and more. For this reason, there is no such thing as an ideal diet that is suited for everyone, just as there is no "magic bullet" that will treat every disease. To ensure that the diet you are following is suited to your needs, it is advisable to work with a nutritionally oriented physician or a certified nutrition specialist—a physician, nutritionist, or chiropractor who has at least a master's degree in nutrition. Such a professional will be able to determine your dietary requirements and discover if you should avoid any foods to which you may unknowingly be allergic or sensitive.

The above discussion mentioned the problem of food allergies and sensitivities. Although this issue is rarely considered or addressed by conventional physicians, it is an important element that must be taken into consideration when creating a healthful diet. Before we discuss it further, however, it should be noted that allergies and sensitivities are not the same thing. A *food allergy* occurs when the immune system reacts adversely to a food ingredient. This type of reaction most commonly affects the mouth and throat, the digestive tract, and the skin. A *food intolerance* or *sensitivity*, on the other hand, does not involve the immune system, but occurs when the body cannot metabolize or digest a food.

It has been found that 90 percent of all food allergies are caused by eight foods: peanuts, tree nuts, milk, eggs, fish, shellfish, soy, and wheat. The most common food intolerance, on the other hand, is lactose intolerance—the inability to digest the sugar found in milk and milk products. Other foods that frequently cause problems include chocolate, corn, and tomatoes and tomato products. However, it should be noted that *any* food has the potential to provoke food allergies and sensitivities, especially if it is eaten on a regular basis.

Some people are made quite ill by the food to which they are allergic or sensitive, causing them to quickly identify the problem food and avoid it in the future. In many cases, though, the person with the allergy or sensitivity has more subtle reactions to the food, and is not aware that it is causing a problem. Sometimes, in fact, people actually crave the food to which they are allergic or sensitive, and feel uncomfortable when that food isn't available, in much the same way that an alcoholic or drug user experiences withdrawal symptoms when deprived of their drink or drug of choice. If you suspect that you suffer from food allergies or sensitivities, we recommend that you seek the help of a physician trained in this area, especially physicians who are members of the American Academy of Environmental Medicine. (For more information, visit their website at www.aaem.com.)

Guidelines for Healthy Eating

Although we recommend that you work with a trained healthcare professional to create the best possible diet—a diet that meets your unique nutritional needs and eliminates any problem foods—it is important that you understand the principles of healthy eating. These principles are really very simple and can be easily incorporated into your lifestyle by following the guidelines presented below:

Eat These Foods as Often as Possible:

❏ Organic whole (unprocessed) foods.

❏ Fresh fruits and vegetables.

❏ Foods rich in essential fatty acids, including cold-water fish such as salmon and sardines, flaxseed, walnuts, and pumpkin seeds.

❏ Fiber-rich foods such as bran and rolled oats.

❏ Foods with a low rating on the glycemic index. (See the inset on page 109.)

Avoid These Foods as Much as Possible:

❏ Refined carbohydrates, such as those found in white bread, pasta made from white flour, white rice, and chips.

❏ Processed "junk" foods.

❏ Sugar, including brown sugar, cane sugar, corn syrup, high-fructose corn syrup, dextrose, fructose, glucose, and maltose.

❏ Saturated fats, trans fatty acids, and hydrogenated oils.

Eat These Foods Only Occasionally:

❏ Salt, caffeine, and alcohol.

You will note that the first guideline in the "eat often" list above is to include organic whole foods in your diet. Whole foods are unprocessed and free of additives and chemicals, such as artificial flavoring, hydrogenated oils, preservatives, and sweeteners. In addition to fresh fruits and vegetables, whole foods include complex carbohydrates such as whole grains and legumes; free-range eggs; free-range meats and poultry that are free of antibiotics and hormones; wild-caught fish, instead of farm-raised fish, which contain antibiotics; and nuts and seeds. All of these foods will provide you with the nutrients you need without including additives that can compromise your health.

As you choose items from the "eat often" list, remember to select a wide variety of foods. This is important because it's an excellent way of obtaining a rich supply of nutrients and fiber. Although you should, of course, steer clear of foods to which you are sensitive or allergic, if you are not lactose intolerant, you can include milk and dairy products such as yogurt and cheese, although we recommend that you choose organic dairy products only. In fact, we don't even want you to avoid oils and fats, although we do recommend that you confine yourself to healthy fats and oils, and that you eat those only in moderation. Excellent food sources for these healthy fats include avocados, nuts, olives, seeds, and wheat germ.

As you can see, for the most part, the "avoid" list focuses on nutrient-poor processed foods such as biscuits, cakes, pasta, white bread, white rice, and various forms of sugar. It also includes hydrogenated oils and trans fatty acids, which are found in many commercially baked goods, including cookies and crackers; many commercial cereals; margarine; and most brands of peanut butter. (Organic nut butters are fine.) At best, the foods on this list provide little or no nutritional value. At worst, they can actually damage your health. The consumption of hydrogenated oils, for instance, has been linked with the development of diabetes, cancer, and cardiovascular disease. For this reason, hydrogenated oils should *never* be eaten. Saturated fats, on the other hand, should be consumed as seldom as possible.

What foods should be consumed only occasionally? Because salt has been linked with a variety of health problems, it is wise to add as little as possible to your foods. While caffeine-containing foods need not be eliminated, you should try to keep your total daily caffeine intake to 200 milligrams or less a day. Finally, you should limit yourself to no more than one or two glasses of red wine per day, avoiding all other alcoholic beverages.

Nutritional Supplementation

As we pointed out in Chapter 1, a healthy diet alone cannot ensure that you receive all of the nutrients your body needs for good health. Therefore, in addition to the SierraSil mineral complex, we

The Low-Glycemic Diet

For years, a low-glycemic diet—a diet low in foods that cause a rapid elevation of sugar and surges of insulin in the bloodstream—was recommended for people with diabetes. But over time, researchers realized that this diet provides benefits for everyone.

Foods recommended on a low-glycemic diet have a low rating on the glycemic index (GI), which ranks carbohydrates according to their effect on blood glucose (sugar). Foods that have a high GI rating elevate blood sugar very quickly. This causes the body to increase its production of insulin, which, in turn, signals the body to store fat, and hinders its absorption of nutrients. On the other hand, foods with a low GI rating help the body maintain normal blood sugar levels; maintain a healthy, fat-burning mode within the body; raise energy levels; enhance mood; improve the body's level of healthy fats; and help control appetite, all the while reducing the risk of chronic degenerative diseases such as diabetes, heart disease, and obesity.

Fortunately, it's easy to enjoy a low-glycemic diet. To start, you'll want to follow these general guidelines:

❑ Eat plenty of fresh, organic fruits and vegetables throughout the day.

❑ Limit your intake of potatoes, as they are a high-glycemic food.

❑ Limit your intake of bread and bread products, eating only small portions of "grainy" breads that include whole grains and seeds. (Look for a product that provides at least 3 grams of fiber per slice.)

❑ Avoid commercial breakfast cereals, which are usually laden with sugar and include hydrogenated fats. Instead, choose breakfast cereals that include organic barley, bran, or oats and are free of hydrogenated fats.

❑ Avoid all sugars, including both granulated sugar and brown sugar.

❑ Bake, grill, or steam your foods, using extra virgin olive oil or coconut oil only sparingly.

❑ Avoid the use of high-fat dressings, gravies, and sauces.

Once you start reaping the benefits of a low-glycemic diet, you'll want to learn more about low-glycemic eating. Websites such as Mendosa.com provide the GI of many common foods and ingredients.

recommend that you supplement your diet with a good multivitamin/multimineral formula. Ideally, the formula you choose should contain the nutrients presented in Table 5.1 in the amounts listed.

TABLE 5.1 RECOMMENDED AMOUNTS OF NUTRIENTS IN MULTIVITAMIN/MULTIMINERAL SUPPLEMENTS	
VITAMIN	**DOSAGE RANGE**
Vitamin A with Beta-Carotene*	5,000 to 25,000 IU
Vitamin B Complex	25 to 300 mg
Vitamin B_{12}**	25 to 500 mcg
Vitamin C	500 to 5,000 mg
Vitamin D_3***	400 to 800 IU
Vitamin E****	400 to 1,200 IU
Vitamin K	80 mcg
Biotin	300 mcg
Choline	25 to 500 mg
Flavonoids	250 to 1,000 mg
Folic Acid	400 to 1,200 mcg
Inositol	25 to 500 mg
PABA	25 to 500 mg
Pantothenic Acid	25 to 500 mg
MINERAL	**DOSAGE RANGE**
Boron	3 to 6 mg
Calcium*****	1,000 to 1,500 mg
Chromium	200 to 600 mcg
Copper	0.5 to 2 mg
Iodine	150 to 300 mcg
Magnesium	400 to 750 mg
Manganese	15 mg

Phosphorus	200 to 400 mg
Potassium	99 to 300 mg
Selenium	100 to 400 mcg
Zinc	22.5 to 50 mg

* Be sure that your beta-carotene is natural, not synthetic. This information is generally provided on the product label.

** Look for vitamin B$_{12}$ in the form of methylcobalamin instead of cyanocobalamin. The methyl form helps maintain circadian rhythms and melatonin, and protects against neural toxicity.

*** Vitamin D$_3$ is the form of vitamin D that can best be used by your body.

**** Be sure that your vitamin E is natural, not synthetic. Natural vitamin E is listed on product labels as d-alpha tocopherol, whereas the synthetic form is listed as dl-alpha tocopherol. Also, when possible, consider taking the complete vitamin E, which contains mixed alpha, beta, delta, and gamma tocopherols and tocotrienols.

***** Take any supplement that contains calcium at least two hours before or after taking SierraSil to ensure the effectiveness of both supplements.

Fortunately, a number of multivitamin/multimineral products on the market provide all of the nutrients listed in Table 5.1, making it easy to get the vitamins and minerals you need for good health. In some cases, though, individuals have nutritional needs that make it necessary to increase their intake of certain nutrients— especially vitamin C, calcium, and magnesium—beyond the amounts provided in multi-nutrient formulas. In such cases, additional supplements must be taken.

Over the years, some of our clients have required nutrients beyond those found in multivitamin/multimineral supplements. In some cases, the clients suffered from higher-than-average levels of stress. In other instances, they were receiving too little sleep, or had been exposed to an unusual number of environmental toxins. When working with these clients, the nutrients listed in Table 5.2 were often helpful in restoring and maintaining good health. Because some of these supplements may not be familiar to you, in addition to supplying the dosage range, we have included a brief explanation of each nutrient's benefits so that you can judge if it warrants further investigation.

TABLE 5.2 RECOMMENDED AMOUNTS OF ADDITIONAL NUTRIENTS

NUTRIENT	DOSAGE RANGE	BENEFITS
Alpha-Lipoic Acid	300 to 600 mg	Helps prevent and treat age-related disorders such as heart disease, diabetes, and the degeneration of the lens and retina of the eye.
Coenzyme Q_{10} (CoQ_{10})	50 to 300 mg	Critical in the production of energy within each human cell, and essential for the health of cells, tissues, and organs.
Fish Oil	1,500 to 3,000 mg	Helps prevent and treat cardiovascular disease, including high blood pressure; has anti-cancer actions; helps relieve the stiffness and swelling of rheumatoid arthritis; and helps control diabetes.
Garlic Extract	200 to 1,200 mg	Reduces total cholesterol while increasing HDLs (good cholesterol), controls high blood pressure, inhibits the development of atherosclerosis, and stimulates blood circulation.
Glutathione	500 to 1,500 mg	Supports the immune system, helps the liver detoxify chemicals, and promotes longevity.
L-Carnitine	2,000 to 4,000 mg	Helps burn unwanted body fat, supports heart health, promotes healthy brain function, and helps detoxify certain drugs.
Lutein	10 to 40 mg	Promotes eye health, reducing the risk of macular degeneration; supports skin health; and may help prevent the thickening of arterial walls.
Lycopene	10 to 20 mg	Reduces the risk of cancer of the breast, colon, prostate, and skin; and may help lower cholesterol levels.
N-Acetylcysteine (NAC)	1,200 to 3,800 mg	Supports the immune system, helps produce healthy new cells, supports the health of the liver and lymphatic system, and helps prevent free radical damage.

Policosanol	10 to 20 mg	Supports the lowering of total cholesterol and LDL-C, and the elevation of HDL-2. Also supports the reduction of vulnerable plaque development.

Water Intake

Water makes up approximately 70 percent of your body, and is the medium through which all of your body's functions occur. Adequate daily water intake is essential for proper brain function, proper transmission of nerve impulses, healthy digestion and metabolism, adequate transport of oxygen to cells and tissues via the bloodstream, healthy kidney and urinary tract function, regulation of body temperature, proper muscle function, and adequate lubrication of joints and tendons. Despite our great need for water, according to the late Dr. F. Batmanghelidj—who spent the last twenty-five years of his life researching water's vital role in optimal health—the vast majority of Americans suffer from chronic dehydration and usually are not aware of it.

Most people do not think they are dehydrated until they experience obvious thirst signals, such as a dry mouth. According to Dr. Batmanghelidj, however, a dry mouth is the *last* outward sign of dehydration. Other, less obvious signs include fatigue, breathing difficulties, sinus congestion, increased susceptibility to infection, and constipation, as well as other gastrointestinal problems. Drinking adequate water throughout the day is a simple way to both prevent and reverse such problems.

Although many people prefer to drink coffee, tea, soda, milk, processed juices, or alcohol to quench their thirst, most of these beverages only increase dehydration by acting as diuretics. That's why we urge you to get in the habit of making water your primary beverage. It is commonly recommended that people drink six to eight glasses of water each day. Remember, though, that herbal teas and fresh fruits and vegetables add to your fluid intake, satisfying some of your body's daily need for water.

Finally, make sure to drink only the purest water available. Avoid tap water, which can contain chlorine, fluoride, and other harmful substances. Instead, drink bottled regular or sparkling mineral water from a company you can trust, or use a high-quality water filter to purify your tap water before drinking it or using it in cooking. The simple addition of high-quality water to your daily diet can pay important dividends in a very short time.

Exercise

Numerous studies have indicated that people who exercise for as little as twenty minutes a day, at least three days a week, live longer and enjoy better health than people who fail to exercise. Although this is hardly news, many people ignore the benefits of regular exercise. The results of this attitude can be seen throughout our society, but most alarmingly, they can be seen in our children, 25 percent of whom are overweight or obese. In addition, research shows that lack of exercise actually worsens arthritis and joint pain, a leading cause of disability among Americans. (For more information on arthritis pain, see the inset on page 115.)

How can you avoid the problems caused by a sedentary lifestyle? By making a commitment to exercise for at least twenty to three minutes, three times a week, you will improve your health by increasing your energy levels, improving blood circulation, decreasing stress, aiding your digestion, improving your sleep, and even enhancing your mental function. Just as important, as you start to notice the overall improvements in your health and appearance, your self-esteem will also be enhanced.

Before beginning an exercise program, we recommend that you consult with your physician. In addition, for best results, you might consider working with a professional fitness trainer for a few weeks so that he or she can guide you in the fundamentals of proper exercise form and technique, and help prevent the injuries that can occur when exercise is done improperly. Professional trainers are especially important if you have any existing health concerns. For instance, if you are already experiencing the pain of arthritis, you should consider water aerobics under the guidance of a professional instructor to minimize wear and tear on your body.

The best exercise programs include a mix of activities that increase muscle strength, flexibility, and aerobic capacity. The building of muscle strength can easily be accomplished by regularly doing push-ups, chin-ups, and sit-ups, or through the use of free weights or weight machines. To improve flexibility, we recommend stretching exercises such as those used in yoga, Pilates, or Tai Chi. For aerobic exercises, consider brisk walking, jogging, bicycling, hiking, and/or swimming. Or you might consider rebounding (jogging or jumping in place on a mini-trampoline). Treadmills, rowing machines, stair climbers, and stationary bikes are other good choices.

In choosing your exercise program, focus on exercises that you find enjoyable. Don't overexert yourself, especially in the beginning. But at the same time, remember the following maxim, which is all too true: If you don't use it, you will indeed lose it!

Sleep and Relaxation

Lack of restful sleep and its inevitable result—fatigue—are per-

The Benefits of Exercise and Weight Loss for Arthritis

Published research shows that losing excess weight can provide significant benefits for people who suffer from arthritis pain, and particularly, for those with osteoarthritis.

In a study published in the July 2005 issue of *Arthritis and Rheumatism,* researchers at North Carolina's Wake Forest University noted that losing a single pound of excess weight results in a four-pound reduction of the joint load placed on arthritic knees while walking. Moreover, in overweight and obese subjects, a 5-percent reduction in excess weight achieved through diet and exercise results in an 18-percent gain in overall physical function.

According to the study's lead researcher, Stephen P. Messier, PhD, "The accumulated reduction in knee load for a one-pound loss in weight would be more than 4,800 pounds per mile walked. For people losing 10 pounds, each knee would be subjected to 48,000 pounds less in compressive load per mile walked." Dr. Messier further noted that weight loss appears to slow the progression of osteoarthritis knee pain.

haps the most common health problems reported by our clients. Due to our busy schedules, we, too, are guilty of not getting enough sleep at times. But we always make it a point to catch up on our sleep as soon as our schedules permit.

The average person requires seven to eight hours of restful sleep each night in order to stay healthy. Unfortunately, studies show that many of us are failing to get that much sleep on a regular basis, and even when we do, we often sleep fitfully and awaken tired and unrefreshed. Over time, lack of sleep can contribute to poor health in a variety of ways. In addition to fatigue, it can compromise your immune function, increasing your susceptibility to disease; diminish your mental function; and increase your risk of harmful accidents.

The failure to get regular periods of relaxation can also be quite harmful. Initially, it can cause stress to accumulate, both physically and emotionally. This, in turn, can cause chronic tension in your muscles, making them less capable of functioning properly. Over time, this can even result in misalignments of the spine, thereby compromising the nerve signals transmitted along the spine to the major organs of the body.

Finally, it's worthwhile to understand the relationship between poor sleep and chronic pain. A benchmark "quality of life" study published by researchers at the University of North Carolina in the *Archives of Family Medicine* (February 17, 2000) released findings that "not being able to sleep with chronic pain is a chief reason that people with arthritis conditions turn to traditional (conventional) and non-traditional (complementary) medical care for relief of their illness." The combination of arthritis pain and sleep loss is often a two-way street. Poor quality of sleep and waking pain create a vicious cycle affecting mood and fatigue levels. The University of North Carolina authors concluded that targeting the total cause of pain is crucial to comfort and recovery.

Tips for Promoting Healthy Sleep

If you suffer from a lack of sleep, you can begin to improve your situation immediately by following a few simple guidelines. First, make a commitment to yourself to go to bed at a time that will allow you to sleep for at least seven hours. Then, make sure that your bedroom is conducive to restful sleep. Keep it clean and free of dust, make sure that it receives adequate fresh air, and keep the temperature at a comfortable level. Also ensure that your mattress is comfortable. Finally, make your bedroom a true sleep area by moving TVs, radios, and/or stereos to another room. If necessary, also eliminate reading materials from your bedroom so that your brain is not overstimulated when you retire for the night. In short, your bedroom should be maintained as your sleeping quarters, not as an entertainment center.

Finally, a few dietary recommendations are in order. It is well known that eating too late in the evening can result in poor sleep. For this reason, we recommend that you avoid eating at least two to three hours before retiring for the night. You might also consider drinking a cup of herbal tea forty-five to sixty minutes before going to bed. Chamomile and valerian root teas are particularly effective in inducing relaxation and sleep.

Tips for Promoting Relaxation

Too many people allow their stress levels to build during the day, causing damage to both their mental and physical health. Fortunately, there are a number of quick and easy ways to promote relaxation even during a busy day. (See the discussion on page 120 to learn about dealing with more severe stress.)

One of the most effective means of promoting relaxation is to simply become aware of your breathing during the day, especially when you are in the midst of activities that can be stressful. During such times, most people have a tendency to take shallow breaths or to even hold their breath. If you notice yourself doing this, take a few minutes to breathe deeply and fully through your belly, ideally with your eyes closed. Once you get in the habit of doing this for a minute or two every half hour or so, you will actually prevent stress from building up.

Another simple yet highly effective relaxation technique is to take a brief break from what you are doing every hour or so. Simply stand up and stretch, breathing deeply and allowing yourself to truly enjoy the stretch. This technique can be especially helpful if you work at a desk all day. If you have time during your lunch break, take a leisurely walk around the block. This, too, is an excellent way to work off stress and recharge your mental batteries.

Creating Healthy Work and Home Environments

Given the increasing levels of environmental toxins in our world, it is important to take any steps necessary to ensure that you live and work in a toxin- and pollutant-free environment. This means ensuring that these environments provide both good-quality air and clean drinking water. Fortunately, it is usually possible to accomplish both of these goals quite easily.

Earlier in the chapter, we discussed the importance of drinking plentiful amounts of pure water each day. (See page 113.) To make sure that the water you drink and use in cooking is as pure as it can be, either buy bottled water from a reliable company, or install a good-quality water filter capable of pulling the impurities out of tap water.

Whether at home or at work, if the air in that area is clean and not overly dry, keep your windows open—weather permitting—to help fresh air circulate throughout the building. To further enhance the quality of your indoor air, we recommend that you place plants throughout your home and, if possible, your place of work. Plants help keep air moist while also enriching it with oxygen. They also act as natural filters, helping eliminate carbon monoxide and organic chemicals.

If weather or unhealthy levels of air pollutants force you to keep windows closed, consider using a negative ion generator to further purify the air inside your home or workspace. Negative ions are air molecules containing an abundance of electrons. The benefit of using a negative ion generator is similar to that of breathing fresh ocean air, which also has a high concentration of negative ions. You will feel energized and more alive. Studies also indicate that the use of a negative ion generator can filter out indoor air pollutants and safeguard against the proliferation of harmful molds and bacteria, thereby improving respiratory function. This is why negative ion generators are especially useful if you work in an air-conditioned building with sealed windows, as this environment often makes it easier for airborne bacteria and fungi to breed, leading to "sick building syndrome."

If the air in your home or work environment tends to be dry, we suggest that you also use a warm-mist humidifier. Ideally, the air you breathe should have a relative humidity of 35 to 55 percent. Breathing air with lower humidity can contribute to respiratory conditions such as sinusitis, and can also exacerbate allergies. Just be sure to clean your humidifier at least once a week so that harmful molds are not allowed to grow inside the machine, and then spread throughout your house.

Another important measure for creating healthier home and work environments is to use people- and pet-friendly materials. This means choosing natural products such as wood, cotton, and metals over synthetic products such as polyester, particle board, and plastics. Certain insulation materials, as well as plywood, should also be avoided because of the formaldehyde they contain. Fortunately, for each synthetic or toxic material or product, there are natural alternatives.

To further improve your home and work environments, take steps to avoid all secondhand smoke and ensure that your furnace filters are efficient. Also reduce any reliance you may have on a coal- or wood-burning stove or fireplace, as both coal and wood emit pollutants as they burn.

It is vital to maintain healthy home and work environments through regular cleanings, and is especially important to regularly clean any carpets or rugs to prevent the buildup of bacteria and mold. Just be careful in your choice of cleaning products, some of which can be toxic to humans, pets, and the environment. Many nontoxic and environment-friendly natural cleaning products are now available. Look for them in health food stores and even in some supermarkets.

Finally, even after you've done all you can to create healthy indoor environments, we recommend that you make it a point to regularly spend time outside in a natural, unpolluted setting, such as a park or your backyard. Most of us spend far too much time indoors, and the consequences of doing so aren't healthy. Take a walk, or simply relax with a book. This is another simple way in which you can improve your health.

IMPROVING MENTAL HEALTH

Many health professionals now believe that 95 percent of all disease is directly due to unresolved stress. That's why mental health is such an important part of the optimal health equation.

If you suffer from anxiety or depression; if you find yourself continually plagued by anger, fear, or grief; or if you have some form of mental illness, such as bipolar disorder, we recommend that you seek competent professional care. The help of a psychiatrist, psychologist, or other professional counselor—or of a physician trained in the field of mind/body medicine—may be just what you need to regain control over your life and your health.

For less serious mental and emotional issues, however, there is much you can do on your own to create feelings of contentment, peace of mind, and positive beliefs and attitudes. The following easy yet effective practices can improve both your mental and physical well-being.

Conscious Breathing

We've already discussed how deep breathing can help alleviate physical stress. By becoming more aware of your breathing patterns and taking deeper, fuller breaths whenever you notice tension building up within you, you can also release feelings of anxiety, anger, fear, and sorrow, as well as increase energy and alertness. Breathing in this manner is sometimes referred to as *conscious breathing* because it involves truly paying attention to your breathing process and to the thoughts and emotions that arise during that process.

Relaxation Exercises

The regular use of relaxation exercises can enable your body to release stored tension, can lighten your mood, and can ultimately allow your mind to return to a natural state of balance. While many different relaxation exercises can be effective, we have found that the following method has been especially helpful to our clients.

Lie down in a comfortable position with your shoes off, at a time when you won't be interrupted. Close your eyes and, starting with your toes, first clench and then relax the muscles in each area of your body. Begin by clenching your toes for a count of "one, two"; then allow them to relax. Repeat the process with your feet, ankles, calves, and thighs, each time clenching the muscles in that region for the prescribed count as you breathe deeply and fully. Continue moving upward along your body, next moving from your buttock and hip muscles to your abdominal muscles, chest muscles, fingers, hands, arms, shoulders, neck, and finally the muscles of your jaw, neck, face, and head. There is no need to strain as you perform this exercise. Simply clench and release each muscle group in turn, allowing the resulting relaxation to flow throughout your body.

Keep in mind that this is only one of many effective relaxation exercises and techniques. To learn additional techniques, visit your local library or bookstore, or perform an Internet search. There, you'll find a wealth of books, tapes, and CDs that can help you relieve stress and enjoy a healthy state of relaxation.

Humor

In the Bible it is written, "A cheerful heart is good medicine." Certainly, the ability to perceive humor and to laugh can be a powerful antidote to tension.

Researchers Robert Ornstein, PhD, and David Sobel, MD, have explored the health benefits of humor, and have found that laughter and a cheerful attitude not only dissipate stress, but also improve immune function. In their book *Healthy Pleasures*, Ornstein and Sobel write, "A robust laugh gives the muscles of your face, shoulders, diaphragm, and abdomen a good workout. . . . The afterglow of a hearty laugh is positively relaxing. Blood pressure may temporarily fall, your muscles go limp, and you bask in a mild euphoria."

The regular experience of laughter and good humor has also been shown to result in an increase in positive attitudes and beliefs. By making a conscious effort to look for the humorous side of life as you go about your normal activities, you will find yourself enjoying each day more fully, and will be far less prone to suffer from stress.

CULTIVATING SPIRITUAL HEALTH

It has been said that all *dis-ease* is ultimately due to feelings of being disconnected from others and God or Spirit. The truth of this observation is borne out by numerous studies which show that people who regularly participate in activities such as prayer, meditation, and worship services typically live longer and healthier lives than people who don't engage in such activities.

Perhaps you already attend services at a place of worship, or perhaps you feel you'd like to begin. If so, you will probably find that this attendance helps you develop greater spiritual health. If, however, you do not choose to engage in formal religious observance, there are other ways in which you can cultivate a healthy spirit.

Prayer

Prayer is the most popular form of spiritual practice in the United States. And over the last few decades, scientific research has confirmed the healing effects of prayer. For example, Larry Dossey, MD, has written extensively about the powerful role prayer can play in helping to heal oneself, one's loved ones, and even strangers. Similarly, colleague Herbert Benson, MD—founding President of the Mind/Body Medical Institute and the Mind/Body Medical Institute Associate Professor of Medicine, Harvard Medical School—has found that praying regularly, or even simply repeating spiritual phrases that invoke God, can produce immediate increases in relaxation and accompanying reductions in stress.

There are many different ways to pray, beginning with the traditional prayers you may have learned growing up. You can also pray by having a personal conversation with God. Or you can simply take time each day to give thanks for the blessings you receive. Many people find that this enhances feelings of joy and contentment and fosters a deeper awareness of the Divine.

To benefit from prayer, choose whatever form feels most appropriate and comfortable for you. Then get in the habit of praying daily.

The Many Benefits of Meditation

In this chapter, we discuss how optimal health is achieved only when you are healthy in body, mind, and spirit. Is there any one practice that can enhance your well-being in all of these areas? The answer is "yes," and the practice is meditation.

The benefits of meditation were first confirmed scientifically during the 1970s. The practice's many positive effects on physical health include improved cardiovascular and immune function, and decreased levels of pain. In fact, the power of meditation is so great that it has been associated with longer life span, better quality of life, and fewer hospitalizations. But meditation also enhances mental health by reducing levels of stress and promoting a sense of calm and well-being. Finally, meditation promotes spiritual health by creating a deeper sense of compassion for and connectedness to others.

Although there are many schools of meditation, including mindfulness meditation, Transcendental Meditation (TM), and Zen, you can also enjoy the rewards of meditation simply by sitting quietly with your eyes closed and focusing your attention on your breathing. As you observe yourself inhaling and exhaling, instead of becoming absorbed by the thoughts and emotions that will automatically arise, allow the thoughts to pass, keeping your attention on your breath. To enhance your meditation practice, you can also mentally repeat a word such as "peace" or "relax" each time you inhale and exhale. Although you may at first find it difficult to sit still for more than a few minutes, with commitment and regular practice, you will be able to meditate for longer and more comfortable periods of time each day. Researchers have found that twenty minutes of meditation practiced twice a day can create lasting improvements in overall health and mood.

Spending Time in Nature

For some people, one of the most direct and visible manifestations of the mystery and sacredness of life is the beauty of nature. Because most of us spend so much time indoors, it is easy to forget that we share this planet with millions of other life forms, all of which are part of the divine circle of life. It is certainly much easier to recognize this fact when you take time to enjoy the outdoors.

There are many ways to experience nature. If you live near the woods or a park, take a walk whenever you can to deepen your connection with the world around you. If you live near the water, take time to watch the waves or the ebb and flow of the tide. Camping, sailing, and canoeing are other ways to connect with nature. Or simply spend time in your garden, tilling the soil and helping plants grow.

By spending more time outdoors, you will soon be better able to recognize the rhythms of life, will appreciate the many wonders this world has to offer, and will feel gratitude that you are part of it. Such feelings can play a powerful role in your efforts to create and maintain optimal health.

CONCLUSION

Most likely, you chose to read this book because you wanted to experience better health, to enjoy more energy, and to rid yourself of pain. By combining the daily use of SierraSil with the health strategies outlined in this chapter, you can significantly improve not only your health, but also the health of your loved ones. Your gains may come slowly at first and initially may not seem significant, but over time, the dividends will become increasingly noticeable and rewarding. The key lies in making these strategies part of your everyday life.

If you are unfamiliar with the recommendations we've outlined throughout this book, you may at first find yourself resisting them or wondering if they will work for you. We can assure you that they will. We know this not only because of the many clients we have seen turn their health around by following the recommendations provided in these pages, but also because of the way in which these strategies have so positively affected our own health. It is our sincere wish that you decide to join us and share in the gift of vibrant health.

Conclusion

For centuries, the earth has shared timely and effective healing gifts with medical science and the people who need them. The willow tree and its bark have given us salicylic acid, the digitalis flower has given us digoxin, and mold has given us penicillin. Within this tradition of targeted and exemplary discoveries comes SierraSil, another healing gift of the earth. A unique mineral compound, SierraSil offers significant supportive relief from the joint pain and discomfort associated with arthritis and other inflammatory conditions. And comfort comes naturally, safely, and quickly—often within just a few days.

Throughout this book, we have diligently shared extensive background information with you about SierraSil, reporting how it was discovered, exploring the natural elements it contains, and relating many impressive personal accounts of its extraordinary pain-relieving results. Most important, because we recognize (and understand) that the best-intended summaries and testimonials are generally met with skepticism and tend to be dismissed as merely anecdotal, we have offered scientific support—compelling statistically significant evidence—focusing on SierraSil's safety and effectiveness. Conducted by an expert team of scientific researchers affiliated with Case Western Reserve University School of Medicine, the extensive battery of clinical tests showed remarkable results in support of SierraSil as a breakthrough natural therapeutic supplement.

Through the practical material we have carefully presented, you should also have a clear understanding of how and why arthritis pain and joint deterioration occurs, as well as how to protect your body from chronic inflammatory responses. By making SierraSil part of your daily health regimen in combination with the self-care recommendations presented in Chapter 5, you can make a healthy difference in your life and the lives of your loved ones.

With the growing amount of scientific information supporting SierraSil's impact on arthritis and chronic inflammatory disease, it's easy to see why we call it the "mineral miracle." If, however, you feel the word "miracle" should be reserved for more divine descriptions, then you can call it a "mineral gift." It really doesn't matter which term you use. What does matter is that if you or someone you know is suffering from inflammatory joint pain, SierraSil can offer effective, safe, timely, and targeted relief. We wish you well on your healing journey.

For more information on the SierraSil mineral complex, including the latest research and studies, visit

www.SierraMountainMinerals.com

Glossary

Absorption. A process by which one substance permeates, or is absorbed by, another substance.

Acute inflammation. *See* Inflammation.

Adsorption. The adhesion of molecules of a gas, liquid, or dissolved substance to a solid surface.

Aerobic. Literally meaning "with oxygen," any activity that involves or improves oxygen consumption by the body.

Aerobic exercise. Any form of exercise that enhances the body's utilization of oxygen. Aerobic exercises include jogging, rebounding, running, swimming, and cycling.

Alternative medicine. A system of medical approaches that do not rely upon drugs, surgery, and other conventional Western medical practices. This type of medical care is also known as complementary health care, holistic medicine, and natural healing.

Amino acid. Any of the over twenty substances used by the body to synthesize proteins.

Antibody. A protein substance produced by the body in response to a specific antigen. Antibodies seek to destroy, weaken, or neutralize the antigen. *See also* Antigen.

Antigen. A bacteria, toxin, foreign blood cell, or other cell that is seen as a threat to the body, and leads to the formation of an antibody. *See also* Antibody.

Antioxidant. Any substance that prevents or slows the process of oxidation. Antioxidant nutrients include vitamins A, C, and E; beta-carotene; coenzyme Q_{10} (CoQ_{10}); selenium; and zinc.

Arteriosclerosis. A chronic condition characterized by thickening, loss of elasticity, and hardening of the arteries, resulting in impaired circulation.

Atherosclerosis. A form of arteriosclerosis characterized by the deposition of plaque on the innermost layer of the artery walls.

Bioaccessibility. The fraction of a substance that is available for absorption by the body.

Bioavailability. The degree to which or rate at which a drug or other substance is absorbed by or becomes available to the body.

Biochemical individuality. A term coined by biochemist Roger Williams, PhD, to describe each person's unique genetic makeup and predisposition, unique metabolism, and specific dietary and nutritional needs.

Boron. A trace mineral that helps maintain healthy bones. Boron aids in calcium metabolism; helps regulate the body's magnesium and phosphorus balance; helps ensure proper function of the endocrine system, which produces and regulates hormones; and improves the body's ability to utilize vitamin D.

Calcium. The most plentiful mineral in the human body. Most of the body's calcium contributes to healthy teeth and bones. The remaining calcium is used in blood clotting, muscle contraction, and nerve transmission; helps regulate cardiovascular function and blood pressure levels; aids in the metabolism of iron; and is required for proper cell division.

Candida albicans. A yeast that naturally occurs in the gastrointestinal tract but, when overgrown, can create a variety of disease symptoms and lead to candidiasis, or systemic yeast infection.

Candidiasis. A chronic and systemic yeast infection caused by the overgrowth of the yeast *Candida albicans*. Also known simply as candida, candidiasis can result in a variety of disease conditions, including allergy, chronic fatigue syndrome, and impaired immunity.

Carcinogen. Any substance, such as an environmental toxin, that can cause cancer.

Carcinogenic. Cancer-causing.

Cartilage. A dense connective tissue found in the joints, rib cage, ears, nose, and throat; and between the intervertebral disks.

Chloride. A macromineral that is an essential part of hydrochloric acid, a vital digestive acid. Chloride also helps regulate the body's acid balance, helps the liver eliminate toxins, and aids in the transport of carbon dioxide to the lungs for excretion.

Cholesterol. A soft waxy substance, found in animal tissues, that is used in the manufacture of hormones, bile acid, and vitamin D. Too much cholesterol, however, can cause fat to build up in artery walls.

Chromium. A trace mineral that is an essential component of glucose tolerance factor (GTF), and is therefore important for proper insulin function, carbohydrate metabolism, and the regulation of blood sugar levels.

Chronic inflammation. *See* Inflammation.

Circulating immune complex (CIC). A substance composed of antigens and antibodies that can become lodged in the body, causing or worsening inflammation. *See also* Antibody; Antigen.

Clay. A fine-grained, firm sedimentary material, often containing an abundance of minerals.

Cobalt. A trace mineral that is a component of vitamin B_{12}. Cobalt plays an essential role in the production of red blood cells and the overall health of other body cells, aids in neuromuscular functions, helps the body produce energy, and contributes to proper digestion.

Collagen. A fiber-like protein that is the main support of skin, tendons, bones, cartilage, and connective tissue.

Copper. A trace mineral that aids in the manufacture of collagen and hemoglobin; is necessary for the synthesis of oxygen in red blood cells; acts as an antioxidant, helping to protect against free radical damage; and helps to increase iron absorption.

C-reactive protein (CRP). A type of protein that is an indicator of inflammation in the body.

Cribbing. A condition in which animals lick or chew on wood and clay to satisfy their craving for the minerals such items contain. In some instances, cribbing also occurs in humans.

EFA. *See* Essential fatty acid.

Electrolyte. Any substance that, in liquid form, is capable of conducting an electric current through the body. Acids, bases, and salts are common forms of electrolytes. Electrolytes help regulate the body's fluid levels, and play a vital role in the transmission of nerve impulses from the brain to the rest of the body.

Environmental illness. An illness caused by exposure to pollutants and toxins in the environment—the air, land, and/or water. Such illnesses can include otherwise unexplained allergies, anxiety and depression, arrhythmia, behavioral problems, chronic fatigue syndrome, eczema and hives, edema, gastrointestinal disorders, headache, muscle ache, respiratory conditions, and sleep disorders.

Environmental toxin. A chemical or other substance released into the environment—the air, land, and/or water—that is hazardous to humans and other animals.

Enzyme. A substance produced by the body and contained in certain foods—primarily fruits and vegetables—that acts as a catalyst for biochemical reactions. Enzymes are necessary for every process the body performs, including breathing, digestion, immune function, reproduction, and organ function, as well as speech, thought, and movement. A certain class of enzymes, known as digestive enzymes, is available as nutritional supplements to assist in the digestion of carbohydrates, fats, fibers, and proteins.

Essential fatty acid (EFA). A fat required by the body's cells to ensure proper cell function. Essential fatty acids cannot be manufactured by the body, and therefore must be supplied by the diet in order to ensure good health. The two primary sources of EFAs are omega-3 fatty acids and omega-6 fatty acids.

Food allergy. An adverse response of the body's immune system to a food. This response most commonly involves the mouth and throat, digestive tract, respiratory system, and/or skin, with symptoms ranging from asthma and eczema to anaphylactic shock.

Food intolerance. A nonallergic adverse response that occurs when the body cannot digest or metabolize a food. Common symptoms range from asthma, diarrhea, and eczema to migraine, depression, and muscle aches.

Free radical. An atom or group of atoms that has at least one unpaired electron, and is therefore unstable. When free radicals occur within the body, they ricochet wildly, damaging cells and contributing to inflammation and the progression of cancer, heart disease, and other disorders. Free radicals naturally occur in the body during energy production, but can also be created in unhealthy amounts by the buildup of toxins and waste products in the body, poor diet, nutritional deficiencies, and exposure to environmental toxins and radiation.

Geophagy. The eating of an earthy substance such as clay, chalk, or earth.

Glucose tolerance factor (GTF). The chemical complex in the body that enhances insulin function.

GTF. *See* Glucose tolerance factor.

HCl. *See* Hydrochloric acid.

Hemoglobin. The iron-containing pigment in red blood cells that carries oxygen.

Hormone. A chemical substance produced in the body that regulates proper cell and organ function, aids in the body's response to stress, and assists in proper metabolism and energy production.

Hydrochloric acid (HCl). An acid secreted by the stomach to activate the digestive enzymes that break food into small particles for absorption.

Immune system. The complex system of organs, tissues, and cells responsible for protecting the body from foreign invaders such as infection and environmental toxins.

Inflammation. An immune system response characterized by redness, swelling, pain, and a feeling of heat. There are two types of inflammation: acute inflammation, which is a short-term response to a wound or an invasion of pathogens or toxins; and chronic inflammation, which is a long-term condition that occurs when the body is unable to resolve a persistent health threat.

Inorganic element. An element that is not composed of organic matter. A mineral is an example of an inorganic element.

Iodine. A trace mineral essential for healthy thyroid function. Iodine also helps regulate metabolism and energy production, and helps ensure that the cells of the body receive enough oxygen.

Iron. A trace mineral whose primary function is the manufacture of hemoglobin. Iron is also necessary for healthy immune function and energy production.

LDL. *See* Low density lipoprotein.

Leaky gut syndrome. A condition that occurs when the intestinal lining becomes overly permeable, allowing undigested food particles and pathogens to move from the gut into the bloodstream, and pathogens outside the gut to enter it.

Lithium. A trace mineral that helps to maintain proper serotonin levels, and thereby helps to stabilize mood, aids in sleep, and promotes brain and nervous system function. Lithium is also involved in immune function.

Low density lipoprotein (LDL). A particle in the blood responsible for depositing cholesterol on artery walls. LDL cholesterol is often referred to as "bad" cholesterol.

Macrominerals. Minerals that constitute 0.01 percent or more of the body's total weight. The macrominerals include calcium, chloride, magnesium, phosphorus, potassium, silicon, sodium, and sulfur.

Magnesium. A macromineral that is involved in hundreds of processes, including the relaxation of muscles, energy production, cell repair and maintenance, nerve transmission, hormone regulation, and the metabolism of proteins and nucleic acids.

Manganese. A trace mineral that is essential for proper brain function and the overall health of the nervous system; helps metabolize proteins and carbohydrates; and is required for cholesterol and fatty acid synthesis, as well as collagen formation.

Metabolism. The biochemical reactions and interactions that take place within the body, resulting in the production of energy and the creation of complex substances that form the material of the tissues and organs.

Mind/body medicine. The field of medicine that studies the interrelationships between thoughts, emotions, attitudes, and beliefs and their ability to create health and disease. Common types of mind/body medicine include biofeedback therapy, cognitive therapy, guided imagery and visualization, hypnosis, and meditation.

Mineral. An inorganic element from the earth—the end product that remains as ash when plant, animal, and human tissues completely decompose following death. Minerals constitute between 4 and 5 percent of the weight of the adult human body, and some minerals are essential to the healthy functioning of the body. *See also* Macrominerals; Trace minerals.

Mitochondria. The cells' internal energy factories. The mitochondria produce energy using a fuel called adenosine triphosphate, a substance synthesized from oxygen and glucose. The mitochondria also play an essential role in all intracellular enzyme activity.

Molybdenum. A trace mineral necessary for the body's proper utilization of iron and the metabolism of carbohydrates.

Neurotransmitter. A biochemical substance that carries signals from one neuron (nerve cell) to another nerve, muscle, organ, or other tissue.

Nickel. A trace mineral that helps in the formation of proteins, is involved in the metabolism of glucose, and plays a role in the breast-feeding process by helping produce the hormone prolactin.

Organic element. An element that is synthesized by plants, animals, and humans. A vitamin is an example of an organic element.

Pathogen. Any microorganism—such as a bacterium, fungus, or virus—capable of causing disease.

Phosphorus. The body's second most abundant mineral, after calcium. Most of the body's phosphorus contributes to healthy teeth and bones. The remaining phosphorus helps form DNA and RNA, catalyzes B-complex vitamins, is involved in cellular communication and numerous enzymatic reactions, helps produce energy, and increases endurance.

Physiology. The collective functions and processes of the body. The term also refers to the branch of biology that deals with the body's functions and processes.

Plaque. A fatty deposit in the lining of a damaged artery, or inside an arterial wall. *See also* Stable plaque; Vulnerable plaque.

Potassium. A macromineral that acts as an electrolyte, or essential body salt, to conduct electric currents throughout the body. Potassium is vital to cellular integrity and fluid balance, plays an important role in nerve function, helps metabolize proteins and carbohydrates, aids in energy production, and helps regulate heartbeat.

Prolactin. A hormone that has many functions, the most significant of which is to stimulate the mammary glands to produce milk.

Relaxation response. A term coined by Herbert Benson, MD, of Harvard Medical School, to describe the physiological effects produced when the body enters a calm state of relaxation as a result of meditation or simply sitting still while focused on one's breathing.

Selenium. A trace mineral that prevents the formation of free radicals, helps maintain a healthy heart, aids liver function, assists in the manufacture of proteins, helps neutralize heavy metals and other toxic substances, and acts as an anti-carcinogen.

Serotonin. A hormone that acts as a "feel good" neurotransmitter in the brain, and influences sleep, mood, and brain functions related to sensory perception.

Silicon. A macromineral that is required for tissue strength and stability; is needed for the health of the bones, skin, hair, and nails; and may play a role in cardiovascular health. Silicon is also considered to be a mineral of detoxification due to its ability to penetrate deep into tissues and aid in the elimination of stored cellular toxins.

Smectite. A form of clay that has healing properties due to its ability to eliminate toxins from the body.

Sodium. A macromineral that helps maintain the body's fluid balance both inside and outside the cells, helps transport carbon dioxide, plays a role in muscle contraction and nerve transmission, is involved in the production of hydrochloric acid, and helps transport amino acids to all the cells of the body.

Stable plaque. A type of plaque that comes from both diet and genetically driven liver synthesis, and forms fatty deposits on the lining of a damaged artery. *See also* Plaque; Vulnerable plaque.

Statin drugs. A class of drugs used to lower blood cholesterol.

Strontium. A trace mineral that works to maintain cell structure and preserve the health of bones and teeth, helping prevent tooth decay and soft bones.

Sulfur. A macromineral that is necessary for collagen formation; is involved in the synthesis of protein; helps maintain the health of hair, skin, and nails; contributes to the process of cellular respiration; is necessary for proper brain function; is vital to the cells' ability to effectively utilize oxygen; and helps protect joint health.

Trace minerals. Minerals that constitute less than 0.01 percent of the body's total weight. The ten officially recognized essential trace minerals include chromium, cobalt, copper, iodine, iron, manganese, molybdenum, selenium, vanadium, and zinc. Additional trace elements considered important to health include boron, lithium, nickel, and strontium.

Vanadium. An essential trace mineral that can help lower cholesterol levels and aid the breakdown and digestion of fats.

Vulnerable plaque. A type of plaque that forms inside artery walls and can rupture, spilling its contents into the bloodstream. *See also* Plaque; Stable plaque.

Zinc. An important trace mineral necessary for over 200 biochemical reactions in the body. Zinc acts as a potent antioxidant and detoxifier; is essential for growth and development, healthy body tissues, the regulation of insulin, proper immune function, and prostate health; plays a vital role in cellular membrane structure and function; and helps maintain adequate levels of vitamin A in the body.

Comparative Mineral Charts

As seen in Chapter 3, according to scientific clinical studies, the safety of the SierraSil mineral complex has been verified in the following lab tests: a 14-Day Acute Oral LD50 Toxicity study, a 90-Day Sub-Acute Oral Toxicity study, an Ames test, and a Dissolution (bioaccessibility) test. There has been zero indication of toxicity from SierraSil to date, even at doses seventy times higher than the recommended daily amounts.

Three human studies, including an internationally registered multi-centered double-blind placebo-controlled clinical study, have also been completed to date.

Of the above-mentioned safety studies, the Sub-Acute Oral Toxicity study in particular demonstrates the nontoxic nature of SierraSil. Sprague-Dawley rats (industry standard for human pharmaceutical testing) were fed up to thirty-five times the equivalent human recommended dose of SierraSil along with their regular diet. All the test animals gained weight and remained healthy. Detailed organ histopathology revealed no areas of concern.

Significantly, at the conclusion of the toxicity testing, a hepatic (liver) analysis of its metal content was conducted. The results showed the iron, lead, arsenic, and aluminum content found in the liver was comparable to placebo-treated controls. In other words, SierraSil did not adversely alter the liver's metal content with this dosing regimen. In summary, the results indicated that iron, lead, arsenic and aluminum were not bioavailable, and that SierraSil was safe for human consumption.

A CLOSER LOOK . . .

In an effort to further support the safety of the SierraSil mineral complex, a number of elements that are contained in its overall composition are discussed in the following section. Within the discussion of each mineral, a table compares the amount contained in a recommended daily dose of SierraSil with the amount found in other common products. As you will see, SierraSil's *bioaccessible* mineral amount (the portion that is accessible to the body) and *bioavailable* amount (the portion that the body actually absorbs) are included in the tables wherever applicable. The bioavailable amounts were determined through the 90-Day Sub-Acute Oral Toxicity study. The bioaccessible amounts were the result of the Dissolution test. If available, the recommended dietary intake (RDI) according to the US Food and Drug Administration are also included. The bioavailability data presented in the following charts is based on extensive toxicology data on rats that were given thirty-five times the recommended human dose of SierraSil.

Aluminum

At 8.2 percent, aluminum is the third most abundant element in the earth's crust.[1] SierraSil contains about 9.4 percent aluminum, which is present primarily as inert minerals—silicates (clays), sulfates, and hydroxides in particular. Although this aluminum content sounds high, only 5.6 percent of this amount (about 0.5 percent of the total) is bioaccessible. The majority forms the basic backbone of the mineral and is nonreactive.[2]

When estimating daily dietary aluminum, 2 to 8 milligrams is considered a low range, while 20 to 40 milligrams is considered high.[3,4] The greatest dietary sources of aluminum are from additives commonly found in baked goods and cheeses. Tea also contains a significant amount of aluminum (up to 1.42 milligrams per gram of dry tea[5]), but this is thought to be less absorbable.[3] Lesser sources of aluminum include drinking water, cooking utensils, and food containers. There is no RDI for aluminum.

SierraSil adds only 13 milligrams of bioaccessible aluminum to the diet at the recommended daily dose.[2] This is a small fraction of the aluminum level found in some antacids, and more than two orders of magnitude below the level of concern found in a general search of medical literature.

When the researchers needed to establish the total mineral content of SierraSil as part of their bioaccessibility testing, they found that some of the silicate minerals were so tightly bound that *aqua regia*, a mix of concentrated nitric and hydrochloric acids and one of the strongest acids available, was not sufficient to release the minerals for assay: "... the problem occurred because silicon could not be fully dissolved by aqua regia in the untreated sample and therefore, the total concentration could not be accurately determined." For this reason, Sierra Mountain Minerals found it necessary to use a *lithium borate fusion method* to completely break down the aluminum silicate matrix and release all of the aluminum and silicate for accurate assay results.

Other dietary factors affect the bioavailability of aluminum. Certain silicates have been shown to chelate aluminum, making it unavailable to the body. SierraSil may contain this type of silicate. Other dietary factors, such as citrates, have been shown to increase the availability of aluminum.[6] SierraSil contains no citrates.

TABLE 1. ALUMINUM SUMMARY	
SOURCE OF ALUMINUM	DIETARY AMOUNT (MILLIGRAMS)
SierraSil (assumed **bioavailable** amount) at daily recommended dose[7]	approximately 0 mg
SierraSil (**bioaccessible** amount) at daily recommended dose[2]	13 mg
Baked goods and cheeses (due to additives)[3,4]	2 to 40 mg
Aluminum-based antacids at maximum daily dose	848 mg

IRON

The earth's crust contains 5.6 percent iron.[1] A recommended daily dose of SierraSil contains about 5.9 percent iron, which is present mostly in jarosite, an iron hydroxide sulfate, and other minerals. The iron in SierraSil is only 2.8 percent bioaccessible, which translates to 3.3 milligrams at the recommended daily dose.[2] This amount is about 18 percent of the FDA's suggested RDI.

TABLE 2. IRON SUMMARY	
SOURCE OF IRON	DIETARY AMOUNT (MILLIGRAMS)
SierraSil (assumed **bioavailable** amount) at daily recommended dose[7]	approximately 0 mg
SierraSil (**bioaccessible** amount) at daily recommended dose[2]	3.3 mg
Prune juice (12 ounces)[8]	7.4 mg
Calves liver (3.5 ounces)[8]	12.4 mg
Chick peas (1 cup)[8]	13.8 mg
FDA Daily recommended dietary intake (RDI)	18 mg

CADMIUM

The amount of cadmium contained in SierraSil is approximately 1.8 parts-per-million (ppm). A recommended daily dose of SierraSil contains 0.09 micrograms (mcg) of cadmium, which is the same as its bioaccessible amount. Chocolate is a significant source of cadmium in the American diet, with common chocolate products containing up to 0.136 parts-per-million (ppm).[9]

TABLE 3. CADMIUM SUMMARY	
SOURCE OF CADMIUM	DIETARY AMOUNT (MICROGRAMS)
SierraSil (**bioaccessible** amount) at recommended daily dose[2]	0.09 mcg
Cigarette (1)[10]	1 to 2 mcg
Chocolate bar (standard 1.5-ounces) with a high cadmium content[9]	5.8 mcg

LEAD

The lead content of SierraSil is about 6.5 parts-per-million (ppm). The amount of lead in a recommended daily dose of SierraSil is 13 micrograms (mcg). However, the bioaccessible amount has been shown to be 0 percent.[2] Chocolate is a significant source of lead in the American diet, with common chocolate products containing up to 0.105 parts-per-million (ppm).[9]

TABLE 4. LEAD SUMMARY	
SOURCE OF LEAD	DIETARY AMOUNT (MICROGRAMS)
SierraSil (assumed **bioavailable** amount) at recommended daily dose[7]	approximately 0 mcg
SierraSil (**bioaccessible** amount) at recommended daily dose[2]	0 mcg
Chocolate bar (standard 1.5-ounces) with a high lead content[9]	4.5 mcg

MERCURY

The amount of mercury found in SierraSil is about 0.58 parts-per-million (ppm). The amount contained in a recommended daily dose of SierraSil is only 1.2 micrograms, of which only 1.4 percent is bioaccessible.[2]

TABLE 5. MERCURY SUMMARY	
SOURCE OF MERCURY	DIETARY AMOUNT (MICROGRAMS)
SierraSil (**bioaccessible** amount) at recommended daily dose[2]	0.009 mcg
Seafood – FDA allowable mercury per 200g serving (1 ppm as methylmercury)	0.19 mcg
Drinking water – FDA allowable mercury per 1L serving (2 ppb)	2 mcg

CHROMIUM

SierraSil contains essentially no chromium VI (hexavalent chromium)—the toxic form. In addition, the chromium contained in SierraSil has been shown to be 0 percent bioaccessible.[2]

ARSENIC

The arsenic contained in SierraSil is about 13 parts-per-million (ppm), of which about 61 percent is bioaccessible.[2] The amount contained in a recommended daily dose of SierraSil is 26 micrograms; the bioaccessible amount is 13 micrograms. This level is too low to determine its speciation or type. Arsenic is a complex element that is difficult to discuss because its toxicity varies widely with type. This has led to misunderstanding in public knowledge about arsenic.

Arsenic trioxide has been used as a medicine for over 2,400 years, and is now FDA approved for the treatment of ADL—a type of leukemia—at doses more than thirty-five times higher than the amount of arsenic found in a recommended daily dose of SierraSil.[11] It is interesting to note that arsenic trioxide is the more toxic *trivalent* form (As^{3+}); SierraSil is likely to contain the less-toxic inorganic *pentavalent* form (As^{5+}). The arsenic in SierraSil is believed to occur in minerals called *arsenates,* which are substantially less toxic that arsenites. Expert opinions suggest it is most likely present as a *ferric arsenate* or as an *arsenate compound* substituting for sulfate in one of the component sulfate minerals.[12] Again, the reason for this speculation is that the level of arsenic in SierraSil is too low to determine its type or speciation.

Adding to the complexity of the arsenic story is that it may have nutrient value. Arsenic is a suspected ultra trace mineral in humans, although no tests have been done to measure arsenic deficiency. However, arsenic deficiency in farm animals has been documented.[13] "Organic arsenic" sometimes occurs at very high levels in seafood, but is widely considered to be much less toxic than inorganic arsenic. This is not relevant to SierraSil.

TABLE 6. ARSENIC SUMMARY	
SOURCE OF ARSENIC	DIETARY AMOUNT (MICROGRAMS)
SierraSil (assumed **bioavailable** amount) at recommended daily dose[7]	approximately 0 mcg
SierraSil (**bioaccessible** amount) at recommended daily dose[2]	13 mcg
Drinking water – FDA allowable arsenic per 1L serving (50 ppb)	50 mcg
Drinking water (US), high level, per 1L serving[14]	190 mcg
Wine – Spanish regulation, 1 mg/L,[15] per 750 mL serving	750 mcg
Arsenic trioxide medication for leukemia[11] (daily dosage)	8,000 mcg

References

1. *CRC Handbook of Chemistry and Physics.* 77th Edition. Boca Raton, FL: CRC Press, 1996.

2. Eickhoff, Curtis and Becalska, Anna. *Dissolution test of SierraSil,* Vizon Scitec, Inc., 2004.

3. PDR*health*: http://www.pdrhealth.com/drug_info/nmdrugprofiles/nutsupdrugs/alu_0020.shtml

4. American Water Works Association: http://www.awwa.org/Advocacy/govtaff/alumipap.cfm

5. Matsushima, F; Meshitsuka, S; Nose, T; and Nippon, Eiseigaku Zasshi. "Contents of aluminum and manganese in tea leaves and tea infusions." October 1993, abstract only, 48(4): 864–72.

6. Jugdaohsingh, et al. "Oligomeric but not monomeric silica prevents aluminum absorption in humans." *American Journal of Clinical Nutrition* (2000) 7: 944–949.

7. "Repeated Dose 90-Day Oral Toxicity Study with 28 day recovery period of SierraSil in Sprague-Dawley Rat." OECD Test No. 408, Vedic Lifesciences, 2004.

8. Whitney, EN and Rolfes, SR. *Understanding Nutrition*, Seventh edition. St. Paul, MN: West Publishing,1996.

9. American Environmental Safety Institute: http://www.aesi.ws/projects/chocolate/index.htm

10. World Health Organization (WHO). Environmental Health Criteria 134, Cadmium International Programme on Chemical Safety (IPCS) Monograph, 1992.

11. Trisenox: http://www.trisenox.com

12. Murray, Haydn. Indiana University, 2004.

13. PDR*health*: http://www.pdrhealth.com/drug_info/nmdrugprofiles/nutsupdrugs/ars_0026.shtml

14. Schoen, Ari; Beck, Barbara; Sharma, Raj; and Dube, Eric. "Arsenic toxicity at low doses: epidemiological and mode of action considerations," *Toxicology and Applied Pharmacology*, 2004.

Bibliography

Chapter 1

Abehsera, Michael. *The Healing Clay.* Secaucus, NJ: Citadel Press, 1979.

Blatt, Harvey; Middleton, Gerald; and Murray, Raymond. *Origin of Sedimentary Rocks.* Englewood Cliffs, NJ: Prentice-Hall, 1972.

David, DR; Epp, MD; and Riordan, H. "Changes in USDA Food Composition Data for 43 Garden Crops, 1950 to 1999." *Journal for the American College of Nutrition* (December 2004) 23: 669–682.

Dorland, WA Newman, editor. *Dorland's Illustrated Medical Dictionary.* Thirtieth edition. Philadelphia: WB Saunders Company, 2003.

Hunter, John M; Horst, Oscar H; and Thomas, Robert N. "Religious Geophagy as a Cottage Industry: The Holy Clay Tablets of Esquipulas, Guatemala." *National Geographic Research Journal* 5, No. 3 (1989) 281–295.

Johns, Timothy and Duquette, Martin. "Detoxification and Mineral Supplementation as Functions of Geophagy." *American Journal of Clinical Nutrition* No. 2 (Feb 1991) 53: 448–456.

Knishinsky, Ran. *The Clay Cure: Natural Healing From the Earth.* Rochester, VT: Healing Arts Press, 1998.

Lieberman, Shari and Bruning, Nancy. *The Real Vitamin & Mineral Book.* Third edition. New York: Avery, 2003.

Trivieri, Larry, Jr., editor. *Alternative Medicine: The Definitive Guide.* Second edition. Berkeley, CA: Celestial Arts/Ten Speed Press, 2002.

Trivieri, Larry, Jr. *The American Holistic Medical Association Guide to Holistic Health.* New York: John Wiley & Sons, 1999.

U.S. Senate Document No. 264. United States Senate. Washington, DC, 1936.

Chapter 2

Angell, Marcia. "Is Academic Medicine for Sale?" *New England Journal of Medicine,* Editorial. No. 20 (May 2000) 342: 1516–1518.

Angell, Marcia. "The Truth About Drug Companies." *The New York Times Review of Books,* Editorial, July 15, 2004.

Angell, Marcia. *The Truth About the Drug Companies: How They Deceive Us and What to Do About It.* New York: Random House, 2005.

Angell, Marcia and Relman, Arnold. S. "Prescription for Profit." *Washington Post,* June 20, 2001.

Cauchon, Dennis. "FDA Advisors Tied to Industry." *USA Today,* September 25, 2000.

Dean, Carolyn. *Death By Modern Medicine.* New York: Nutrition Institute of America, 2003.

Fletcher, RH and Fairfield, KM. "Vitamins for Chronic Disease Prevention in Adults: Clinical Applications." *JAMA* (June 2002) 287: 3127–3129.

Garrison, Robert and Somer, Elizabeth. *The Nutrition Desk Reference.* Third edition. New Canaan, CT: Keats Publishing, 1995.

Graham, David J. Testimony Before US Senate Finance Committee, November 18, 2004.

"Harvard Researchers Publish JAMA Articles Recommending Vitamin Supplements for All Adults." Press Release. Council for Responsible Nutrition, Washington, DC. June 20, 2002.

Lazarou, J; Pomeranz, BH; and Corey, PN. "Incidence of Adverse Drug Reactions in Hospitalized Patients: A Meta-Analysis of Prospective Studies." *JAMA* (November 25, 1998) 279: 1200–1205.

Lieberman, Shari and Bruning, Nancy. *The Real Vitamin & Mineral Book.* Third edition. New York: Avery, 2003.

Murray, Haydn. Personal correspondence to Michael Bentley, Sierra Mountain Minerals, Inc., April 30, 2004.

Pauling, Linus. *How to Live Longer and Feel Better.* New York: W.H. Freeman, 1986.

Pauling, Linus. Interview by Larry Trivieri, Jr., April 1993.

Rubin, Rita. "FDA Whistleblower Claims He'll Be Forced From Post." *USA Today,* November 25, 2004.

Starfield, Barbara. "Is US Health Really the Best in the World?" *JAMA* No. 4 (July 26, 2000) 284: 2184–2185.

Tansey, Bernadette. "Hard Sell: How Marketing Drives the Pharmaceutical Industry." *San Francisco Chronicle,* February 27, 2005.

Trivieri, Larry, Jr., editor. *Alternative Medicine: The Definitive Guide.* Second edition. Berkeley, CA: Celestial Arts / Ten Speed Press, 2002.

Trivieri, Larry, Jr. *The American Holistic Medical Association Guide to Holistic Health.* New York: John Wiley & Sons, 1999.

Tufts, A. "Only 6% of Drug Advertising Material Is Supported by Evidence." *British Medical Journal* No. 7438 (February 28, 2005) 328: 485.

2005 Reporter's Handbook for the Prescription Drug Industry. Washington, DC: Pharmaceutical Research and Manufacturers of America (PhRMA), 2005.

Venturi, Ken. Testimony Before the US House Subcommittee on Human Rights and Wellness, September 21, 2004.

Chapter 3

Forman, JP; Stampfer, MJ; and Curhan, GC. "Non-Narcotic Analgesic Dose and Risk of Incident Hypertension in US Women." *Hypertension* (September 2005) 46: 500–507.

Graham, David J. Testimony Before US Senate Finance Committee, November 18, 2004.

Maugh, Thomas H, II. "Study Sees Painkiller Risk for Women." *Los Angeles Times,* August 16, 2005.

Merck Manual of Medical Information. Second edition. Whitehouse Station, NJ: Merck Research Laboratories, 2003.

Miller, MJS; Ahmed, S; Bobrowski, P; and Haqqi, T. "Suppression of Human Cartilage Degradation and Chondrocyte Activation by a Unique Mineral Supplement (SierraSil) and a Cat's Claw Extract, Vincaria." *JANA* No. 2 (2004) 7: 32–39.

Piscoya, J; Miller, MJS; et al. "Efficacy and Safety of Freeze-Dried Cat's Claw in Osteoarthritis of the Knee: Mechanisms of Action of the Species *Uncaria guianensis.*" *Inflammation Research* (2001) 50: 442–448.

"Repeated Dose 90-Day Oral Toxicity Study with 28 Day Recovery Period of SierraSil in Sprague Dawley Rat." OECD Test No. 408, Vedic Lifesciences, 2004.

Singh Gurkirpal. "Recent Considerations in Nonsteroidal Anti-Inflammatory Drug Gastropathy." *The American Journal of Medicine*, July 27, 1998.

Taylor, Leslie. *The Healing Power of Rainforest Herbs.* Garden City Park, NY: Square One Publishers, 2005.

Chapter 4

American Heart Association. "Inflammation, Heart Disease, and Stroke: The Role of C-Reactive Protein." Fact Sheet, 2005.

Appleton, Nancy. *Stopping Inflammation: Relieving the Cause of Degenerative Diseases.* Garden City Park, NY: Square One Publishers, 2005.

"C-Reactive Protein as a Heart Disease Risk Factor." *The Doctor's Prescription for Healthy Living* (January 1999) 4: 1.

Fichtlscherer, S, et al. "Elevated C-Reactive Protein Levels and Impaired Endothelial Vasoreactivity in Patients With Coronary Artery Disease." *Circulation* No. 9 (2000) 102: 1000.

Fuster, Valentin, editor. *The Vulnerable Artherosclerotic Plaque: Understanding, Identification and Modification.* New York: Blackwell Publishing, 2002.

Moss, Ralph. "The War on Cancer." *Townsend Letter for Doctors and Patients* (November 2001) 220: 22–23.

Rifai, N and Ridker, PM. "Inflammatory Markers and Coronary Heart Disease." *Current Opinion in Lipidology* No. 4 (August 2002) 88: 554–567.

O'Byrne, KJ and Dalgleish, AG. "Chronic Immune Activation and Inflammation as the Cause of Malignancy." *British Cancer Journal* No. 4 (August 17, 2001) 85: 473–483.

Sinatra, Stephen. *Coenzyme Q10 and the Heart.* Chicago: McGraw-Hill, 1999.

Sinatra, Stephen. *The Coenzyme Q10 Phenomenon.* Chicago: McGraw-Hill, 1998.

Sinatra, Stephen. *Lower Your Blood Pressure in Eight Weeks: A Revolutionary Program for a Longer, Healthier Life.* New York: Ballantine Books, 2003.

Sinatra, Stephen. *The Sinatra Solution: New Hope for Preventing and Treating Heart Disease.* Chicago: Basic Books, 2005.

Tomasi, S, et al. "High C-Reactive Protein Level May Be a Marker for Cardiac Events." *American Journal of Cardiology* (June 15, 1999) 83: 1595–1599.

Ventura, HO. "Rudolph Virchow and Cellular Pathology." *Clinical Cardiology* (July 2000) 23 (7): 550.

Young, JL and Libby, P. "Cytokines in the Pathogenesis of Atherosclerosis." *Journal of Thrombosis and Haemostasis* No. 4 (October 2002) 88: 554–567.

Chapter 5

Batmanghelidj, F. *Your Body's Many Cries for Water.* Falls Church, VA: Global Health Solutions, Inc., 1992.

Benson, Herbert. *The Relaxation Response.* New York: HarperTorch, 1976.

D'Adamo, Peter and Whitney, Catherine. *Eat Right 4 Your Type.* New York: GP Putnam's Sons, 1996.

Ivkers, Robert; Anderson, Robert; and Trivieri, Larry, Jr. *The Complete Self-Care Guide to Holistic Medicine.* New York: Tarcher/Putnam, 1999.

Lieberman, Shari and Bruning, Nancy. *Dare to Lose.* New York: Avery, 2002.

Lieberman, Shari and Bruning, Nancy. *The Real Vitamin & Mineral Book.* Third edition. New York: Avery, 2003.

Sinatra, Stephen. *Coenzyme Q10 and the Heart.* Chicago: McGraw-Hill, 1999.

Sinatra, Stephen. *The Coenzyme Q10 Phenomenon.* Chicago: McGraw-Hill, 1998.

Sinatra, Stephen. *Lower Your Blood Pressure in Eight Weeks: A Revolu-*

tionary Program for a Longer, Healthier Life. New York: Ballantine Books, 2003.

Sinatra, Stephen. *The Sinatra Solution: New Hope for Preventing and Treating Heart Disease*. Chicago: Basic Books, 2005.

Trivieri, Larry, Jr., editor. *Alternative Medicine: The Definitive Guide*. Second edition. Berkeley, CA: Celestial Arts/Ten Speed Press, 2002.

Trivieri, Larry, Jr. *The American Holistic Medical Association Guide to Holistic Health*. New York: John Wiley & Sons, 1999.

Wolcott, William and Fahey, Trish. *The Metabolic Typing Diet*. New York: Doubleday, 2000.

About the Authors

Dr. Shari Lieberman earned her PhD in Clinical Nutrition and Exercise Physiology from The Union Institute, Cincinnati, Ohio, and her Master of Science degree in Nutrition, Food Science and Dietetics from New York University. She is a Certified Nutrition Specialist (CNS); a Fellow of the American College of Nutrition (FACN); a member of the New York Academy of Science and the American Academy of Anti-Aging Medicine (A4M); a former officer and present board member of the Certification Board for Nutrition Specialists; and President of the American Association for Health Freedom. She is the recipient of the National Nutritional Foods Association 2003 Clinician of the Year Award and a member of the Nutrition Team for the New York City Marathon. Dr. Lieberman is the author of the best-selling *The Real Vitamin & Mineral Book; User's Guide to Brain-Boosting Supplements; Dare to Lose: 4 Simple Steps to a Better Body; Get Off the Menopause Roller Coaster; Maitake Mushroom and D-fraction; Maitake King of Mushrooms;* and *All About Vitamin C.*

Dr. Lieberman is also the Founding Dean of New York Chiropractic College's MS Degree in Clinical Nutrition, contributing editor to the American Medical Associations' 5th Edition of *Drug Evaluations,* peer reviewer for scientific publications, published scientific researcher, and presenter at numerous scientific conferences. A frequent guest on television and radio programs as an authority on nutrition, Dr. Lieberman has been in private practice as a clinical nutritionist for over twenty years. You can visit her website at *www.drshari.net.*

Dr. Alan Xenakis earned dual doctorates in Medicine and Applied Science from Boston University School of Medicine, and master's degrees in Public Health and Health Dynamics from Harvard University and Sargent College of Allied Health. He also holds degrees in Chemistry from the University of New Hampshire, Master of Science from Boston University, Master of Public Health from Harvard University, Doctor of Science from Boston University, and Doctor of Medicine from Boston University.

A renaissance leader in the delivery of integrative healthcare solutions for physicians and their patients, Dr. Xenakis's professional career spans medical center research, university teaching, healthcare management consulting, and private and public company executive management. He is the founder of XenaCare—a national company providing integrative healthcare education, clinical evaluation, and access to proprietary therapeutic non-prescription pharmaceuticals to board certified practicing medical physicians and their patients.

Dr. Xenakis is the author of *Why Doesn't My Funny Bone Make Me Laugh,* and has published in peer review journals, including *The American Heart Journal, Journal of Physiology,* and *IEEE Transactions of Biomedical Engineering.* His features have appeared in *Pharmacy Times, Drug Store News,* and *The Cortlandt Forum.* He has also collaborated or lectured with leading healthcare groups, including The American Heart Association, The American College of Sports Medicine, The Massachusetts College of Pharmacy, The American Cancer Society, The American Medical Association, The Joslin Diabetes Center, The Framingham Heart Group, The Food and Drug Administration, The Environmental Protection Agency, The American Association of Pharmaceutical Scientists, The American Arthritis Foundation, and The American College of Allergy and Immunology.

Dr. Xenakis has served as a national television and radio program producer, reporter, and anchor, appearing on major network, public, and cable television. He is an "Emmy" winner and the recipient of numerous domestic and international awards. You can visit his website at *www.Xenacare.com.*

Index

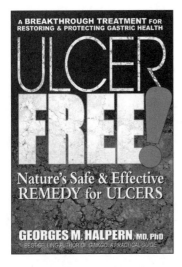

A BREAKTHROUGH TREATMENT FOR
RESTORING & PROTECTING GASTRIC HEALTH

Nature's Safe & Effective
REMEDY for ULCERS

GEORGES M. HALPERN, MD, PhD
BEST-SELLING AUTHOR OF GINKGO: A PRACTICAL GUIDE

ULCER FREE!
Nature's Safe and Effective Remedy for Ulcers
Georges M. Halpern, MD

Over 4 million Americans are diagnosed annually with peptic ulcer disease. Many learn to live with the resulting heartburn, acid reflux, nausea, gas, and stomach pain with the help of over-the-counter antacids. These products may stop the pain, but only temporarily. Furthermore, the underlying condition can worsen. But it doesn't have to be that way. *Ulcer Free!* is a practical guide to understanding the causes of and effective treatments for peptic ulcer disease.

The book begins with a look at why we get ulcers. It examines the *Helicobacter pylori* bacterium—the culprit behind the majority of stomach ulcers. It also discusses the growing number of ulcers caused by NSAIDs—over-the-counter pain relievers, more commonly known as aspirin, ibuprofen, naproxen, and a variety of other products. The book then offers an unbiased look at the treatments—conventional and alternative—that can stop the symptoms of and actually heal ulcers. Finally, *Ulcer Free!* introduces the breakthrough nutrient Zinc-Carnosine, which can be used in conjunction with other treatments or on its own.

If you are tired of being victim to continual gastric distress, *Ulcer Free!* can help. Up-to-date and accurate, it offers the key to permanent relief.

Georges M. Halpern, MD, attended medical school at the University of Paris, France. He subsequently received a PhD from the Faculty of Pharmacy, University of Paris XI—Chatenay Malabry. A Fellow of the American Academy of Allergy and Immunology, Dr. Halpern is board certified in internal medicine and allergy, and is Professor Emeritus of Medicine at the University of California—Davis. He is also a Distinguished Professor of Medicine at the University of Hong Kong.

$14.95 • 208 pages • 6 x 9-inch quality paperback • ISBN 0-7570-0253-6

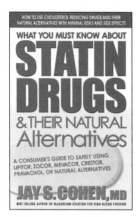

WHAT YOU MUST KNOW ABOUT STATIN DRUGS & THEIR NATURAL ALTERNATIVES

Jay S. Cohen, MD

Over 100 million Americans suffer from elevated cholesterol and C-reactive proteins—markers that are linked to heart attack, stroke, and other cardiovascular disorders. Here is a guide that explains the problems caused by statins, and offers easy-to-follow strategies that will allow you to benefit from these drugs while avoiding their side effects. The author also provides natural alternatives that have proven effective in lowering cholesterol.

If you have elevated cholesterol and C-reactive proteins, or if you are now using a statin, *What You Must Know About Statin Drugs & Their Natural Alternatives* can make a profound difference in the quality of your life.

$15.95 • 224 pages • 6 x 9-inch quality paperback • ISBN 0-7570-0257-9

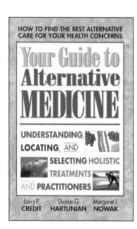

YOUR GUIDE TO ALTERNATIVE MEDICINE

Understanding, Locating, and Selecting Holistic Treatments and Practitioners

Larry P. Credit, Sharon G. Hartunian, and Margaret J. Nowak

This comprehensive reference clearly explains alternative approaches to numerous health disorders in an easy-to-read format. For every complementary care option discussed, there is a description and brief history; a list of conditions that respond; an explanation of how the therapy works; a directory of professional organizations that can offer you further information; information on the cost and duration of treatment; a discussion of what you should expect regarding the credentials and educational background of practitioners; recommended readings; and more. To find those therapies most appropriate for a specific condition, there is even a unique troubleshooting chart that lists common disorders along with the complementary approaches best suited to treat them.

$11.95 • 208 pages • 6 x 9-inch quality paperback • ISBN 0-7570-0125-4

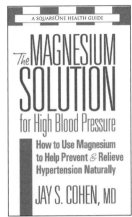

THE MAGNESIUM SOLUTION FOR HIGH BLOOD PRESSURE

How to Use Magnesium to Help Prevent and Relieve Hypertension Naturally

Jay S. Cohen, MD

Approximately 50 percent of all Americans have hypertension, a devastating disease that can lead to hardening of the arteries, heart attack, and stroke. While many medications are available to combat this condition, these drugs come with potentially dangerous side effects. When Dr. Jay S. Cohen learned of his own vascular condition, he was well aware of the risks associated with standard treatments. Based upon his research, he selected a safer option—magnesium.

In *The Magnesium Solution for High Blood Pressure,* Dr. Cohen describes the most effective types of magnesium for treating hypertension, explores appropriate magnesium dosage, and details the use of magnesium in conjunction with hypertension meds. Here is a proven remedy for anyone looking for a safe, effective approach to the treatment of high blood pressure.

$5.95 • 96 pages • 4 x 7-inch mass paperback • ISBN 0-7570-0255-2

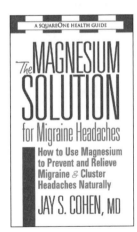

THE MAGNESIUM SOLUTION FOR MIGRAINE HEADACHES

How to Use Magnesium to Prevent and Relieve Migraine and Cluster Headaches Naturally

Jay S. Cohen, MD

More than 30 million people across North America suffer from migraine headaches. Over the years, a number of drugs have been developed to treat migraines, but these treatments don't work for everyone, and come with a high risk of side effects. Fortunately, Dr. Jay S. Cohen has discovered an alternative—magnesium.

This easy-to-understand guide explains what a migraine is, and shows how magnesium can play a key role in preventing and treating migraine headaches. It also describes what type of magnesium works best, and how much magnesium should be taken to prevent or stop migraines. For those who are looking for a safe and effective approach to the prevention and treatment of migraine and cluster headaches, Dr. Cohen prescribes a proven natural remedy in *The Magnesium Solution for Migraine Headaches.*

$5.95 • 96 pages • 4 x 7-inch mass paperback • ISBN 0-7570-0256-0

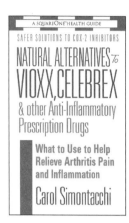

Natural Alternatives to Vioxx, Celebrex, & Other Anti-Inflammatory Prescription Drugs

What to Use to Help Relieve Arthritis Pain and Inflammation

Carol Simontacchi

Beyond today's headlines and pharmaceutical spin is an underlying truth—COX-2 inhibitor drugs can be extremely dangerous to your health. While these drugs do relieve pain and inflammation, the potential for heart attack and stroke has proven too great a risk for many. For those who are looking for other options, health expert Carol Simontacchi has created a guide to using safer natural alternatives. Written in easy-to-understand language, this book provides solid information about nature's most effective treatments.

The book begins by examining the causes of pain and inflammation, and then looks at both pharmaceutical and holistic approaches to dealing with this condition. What follows is a concise discussion of the most effective natural supplements available, including bromelain, cat's claw, curcumin, fish oil, ginger root, glucosamine and chondroitin, anti-inflammatory minerals, and SierraSil. Each supplement is examined for its method of action, scientific documentation, and proper dosage. The author has even included an anti-inflammatory menu plan and a selection of healthful recipes.

Although natural product companies may not have the advertising dollars enjoyed by the pharmaceutical industry, the beneficial effects of natural remedies should not be overlooked. *Natural Alternatives to Vioxx, Celebrex & Other Anti-Inflammatory Prescription Drugs* provides a vital resource for those in search of a safer solution.

Carol Simontacchi, CCN, MS, is a certified clinical nutritionist and the author of a number of books on nutrition, including *Your Fat Is Not Your Fault, The Crazy Makers,* and *A Woman's Guide to a Healthy Heart.* In addition, Ms. Simontacchi is a highly sought-after lecturer who speaks to professional and lay audiences across the country on important health topics. She has appeared on numerous national, regional, and local radio and TV shows, and her work has been featured in *Newsday, First for Women, Woman's Day,* and other popular publications.

$5.95 • 128 pages • 4 x 7-inch mass paperback • ISBN 0-7570-0278-1

For more information about our books, visit our website at www.squareonepublishers.com